Clinical Mentation Evalu

Michael Hoffmann

Clinical Mentation Evaluation

A Connectomal Approach to Rapid
and Comprehensive Assessment

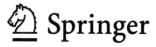 Springer

Michael Hoffmann, MD, PhD
Professor of Neurology
University of Central Florida
Chief of Neurology
Orlando VA Medical Center
Orlando, FL
USA

ISBN 978-3-030-46323-6   ISBN 978-3-030-46324-3   (eBook)
https://doi.org/10.1007/978-3-030-46324-3

This Springer imprint is published by the registered company Springer Nature Switzerland AG
The registered company address is: Gewerbestrasse 11, 6330 Cham, Switzerland

For Bronwyn, Jenna Leigh, and Michael

Notice to the Readers

Medicine, both as a science and art, is a field that is undergoing constant and increasingly rapid changes. These include changes in the treatment of diseases and conditions that include not only drug treatment but also other types of managements, including device therapies. The author of this book, together with Springer Publishing Company, has reviewed the sources of the information, referenced in this book, for accuracy and reliability. Because of the rapid change of knowledge inherent in medicine and the ever-present chance of human error, the author and publisher cannot mandate that all information is completely accurate and comprehensive in scope. The readers are encouraged always to check the information gleaned from this book and compare to other reliable authorities and sources. This should include product information from pharmaceutical companies, when medications are concerned, and checking particular practices with their local physician groups as these can vary across cultures and countries.

Acknowledgments

The evolution of my thinking and ultimately this book is tribute to many friends and colleagues that helped me in my formative years. I was very fortunate to have Professor Phillip Tobias as my Anatomy Professor and Dean of the medical school at the University of Witwatersrand. He taught us human anatomy from not one, but three large books called *Man's Anatomy* part 1, 2, and 3 but more importantly enkindled in his students a fascination for human origins that he was so famous for. Professors Pierre Bill and John Cosnett of the University of Kwa-Zulu Natal, Durban, for their patient and expert teaching in clinical neurology, guiding my early career development. Professor John Robbs, Head of Surgery and Vascular Surgery, University of Kwa-Zulu Natal, Durban, for his enthusiastic support and promotion of my early forays into cerebrovascular medicine and helping form the Durban Cerebrovascular Group. Professor Bill Pryse-Phillips helped land my first neurology job at Memorial University, Canada, while he researched and wrote his book, *Neurology Dictionary*. Professors JP Mohr and Ralph Sacco enthusiastically guided me through my stroke fellowship and instilled the fervor for computerized registry analyses at Columbia University, New York. I am very fortunate to have the continued guidance and mentorship in cognitive neurology and cognitive neuroscience from Professor Frederick Schmitt of the Sanders Brown Aging Institute at the University of Kentucky and Professor Ken Heilman of University of Florida. I am grateful to Dr Fiona Crawford and Dr Michael Mullen for providing me with a platform for launching neuro-archeological seminars at the Roskamp Institute in Sarasota and promoting clinical cognitive neurology to flourish side by side with their high-level neuroscience research.

Registry data used

Clinical examples and radiological images were sampled from the following IRB approved registries of which MH is the principal investigator. These registries pertained to the collection of clinical investigation, radiological and management data of consecutive stroke and cognitive impairment patients, aged 18-90 years were accrued through prospectively coded dedicated stroke and cognitive disorders registries in tertiary referral centers. These were approved by the relevant University Institutional Review Boards and the latter three registries were also in compliance with HIPAA (Health Insurance Portability and Accountability Act) regulations when this was enacted.

Clinical stroke registries and cognitive registries referenced

1.   The NIH-NINDS Stroke Data Bank (New York)
Under the following contracts; N01-NS 2-2302, N01-NS-2-2384, N01-NS-2-2398, N01-NS-2-2399, N01-NS-6-2305
Status: Stroke research fellow (1990–1991)

2.   The Durban Stroke Data Bank. University of KwaZulu-Natal, Durban
South Africa (approved by the Ethics Board of the University of KwaZulu-Natal)
Status: Principal Investigator (1992–1998)

3.   The USF-TGH Stroke Registry. IRB # 102354 (University of South Florida)
Status: Principal Investigator (2002–2020)

4.   The USF-Cognitive Stroke Registry. IRB # 106113 (University of South Florida)
Status: Principal Investigator (2007–2020)

5.   Frontotemporal lobe disorders and related war illness retrospective analysis (OVAMC)
Status: Principal Investigator (April 2020 to present)

Contents

Chapter 1
Introduction: Overview and Challenges of Cognitive and Behavioral Assessment

Through the collection of extensive amounts of computerized clinical and investigative information, I have always valued the data-driven approach that can be derived from registries. It is a more accurate method that can be viewed as a way of spawning hypotheses that are more likely to be worth investigating further, rather than hypotheses based primarily on intuition. What follows is hypothesis-driven research. Through the biological model of stroke, I have studied the type and nature of cognition in stroke through four separate digitized cognitive stroke registries in a sojourn through six different academic centers in three different countries (South Africa, USA, Canada). Stroke patients are particularly instructive as the deficits present relatively suddenly; they are frequently dramatic (imitation behavior, anosognosia) yet often resolve spontaneously. The inordinately rich nature of cognitive and behavior impairment syndromes, conjure up both a fascination of brain functioning but also have important treatment and management consequences for clinical brain disorders. For example, it has long confounded clinicians that the almost universally successful animal studies in stroke have all failed in humans without exception. This is despite over several decades worth of clinical trials in cerebrovascular disease. My own firm conviction, based on the research of these aforementioned digitized registries, is that our rudimentary and often nonexistent documentation of higher cortical functions in stroke is to blame. We know that approximately 90% of the brain has to do with higher order cognitive function, yet we pay penurious attention to these capacities in our clinics and in human clinical trials.

Why Is This Important?

1. Mental status abnormalities are present in most if not all neurological disorders (vulnerable hub hypothesis) [1] (Fig. 1.1).
2. About 50–78% of people with mild cognitive impairment (MCI) are not diagnosed in primary care populations [2].

© Springer Nature Switzerland AG 2020
M. Hoffmann, *Clinical Mentation Evaluation*,
https://doi.org/10.1007/978-3-030-46324-3_1

Brain Disorders

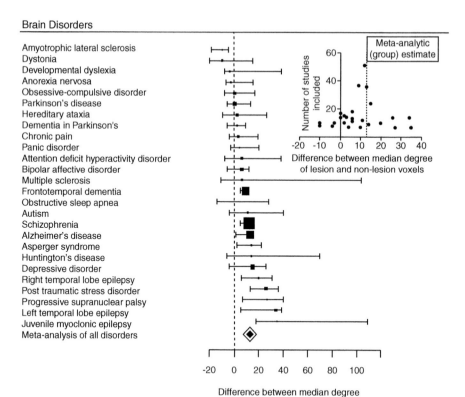

Fig. 1.1 Mental status abnormalities are present in most if not all neurological disorders [1]. Box plot of 26 neurological disorders, depicting the difference in median degree of lesion voxels versus non-lesion voxels (95% CI) with the size of the box being proportional to number of MRI studies published. The insert on the right shows the relationship between sample size versus the difference in median degree for all studies

3. They are the most important abilities for patients and hence the most important part of the examination.
4. Increasingly there is an appreciation that many cognitive deficits including dementias may be reversible [3–5].

The Need for a Flexible Time-Based Approach

The challenge nowadays with neurological syndrome presentations is no longer merely lesion localization, but the degree, extent, and nature of a cognitive and/or behavioral impairment. Increasingly, neurological disorder management has become more emergent: stroke, status epilepticus, fulminant headache syndromes, meningitis, and autoimmune encephalitis spectrum of disorders. These have protocols that are quality management controlled by our various institutions, requiring, rapid, time-based assessments which always includes a brain scan. The constraints of "time is brain" (stroke) and "time is limited" (dementia) both dictate a time-based cognitive testing approach. To benefit from all the varying clinical neuroscience knowledge bases, the testing methodology also needs to encompass a cross disciplinary multi-tiered approach, while using a time-based battery of tests that may range from just a few minutes to several hours. Special relevance to frontal network syndromes (FNS) testing in particular is advocated. This relates to the expansive frontal network that is viewed as a supervisory and wide-ranging cognitive system (metacognition). Hence, evaluation of FNS may be the most sensitive indicator of overall cognitive status.

A system of cognitive and behavioral diagnostic tests is required that are tiered as well as context appropriate for diagnosing mental status. Such an approach needs to incorporate behavioral neurological, neuropsychiatric, and neuropsychological components and be based on the newly appreciated intrinsic brain networks. The most important and pervasive cognitive processes, frontal network syndromes (FNS), are ubiquitous in neurological and psychiatric disease, yet measurement remains poor with few available tests. The two most commonly, clinically employed tests: (1) the Mini Mental State Examination (MMSE) does not even measure frontal systems and (2) the Montreal Cognitive Assessment (MOCA) samples some cognitive aspects but not frontal behavioral domains. Hence, there exists a dilemma between the need for accurate clinical frontal network system assessment and the current battery of tests available for this purpose. Clinical cerebrovascular and neurological decision-making for example, is severely constrained by a 4.5 h so called thrombolytic therapy window. During a typical stroke, approximately 2 million neurons and 14 billion synapses are lost each minute [6]. In the setting of multiple concurrent investigations including neuroimaging, laboratory and cardiac investigations, mentation assessment is taxing. In such an emergency evaluation, time allotment of only a few minutes is left for clinical assessment of the patient, and in the emergent setting, there is no place for formal neuropsychological assessment. Common clinical experience in cognitive impairment and dementia evaluation is challenging from another perspective. The degree of cooperation, inattention, abulia, and restlessness of many patients may leave only a few minutes for testing at best. Historically and philosophically, testing of the higher cortical brain functions has been approached differently by the three major disciplines (Neurology, Psychiatry, Neuropsychology) concerned with assessment of behavioral and cognitive effects of brain lesions and conditions. Each has different "cultures" and approaches to this clinical challenge, but because each has unique contributions, they complement each other. These consist of (i) behavioral neurological approach comprising a myriad of syndromes that are best described in ordinal and nominal data terms, (ii) neuropsychiatric approach with syndromes described in terms of prespecified criteria (DSM-V) and configured to nominal data, and (iii) neuropsychological battery approach almost exclusively described according to numerical data and compared to normative data, less often ordinal and nominal data.

Not only time is limited by the frequently encountered patient who cannot cooperate adequately for more than a few minutes but also time constraints are severely limited for most if not all busy clinicians. Aside from emergency-room neurological patients, it is common place in a routine clinic to be assigned no more than 45–60 min for a "new" patient. Given the number of activities that have to be compressed into this time frame (history and physical, laboratory and neuroimaging ordering or reviewing, counseling, medication, and treatment strategies), this leaves at best no more than 10–15 min for an assessment of the vast panoply of human higher cortical functions – a tall order indeed!

Research emanating from cognitive stroke registries revealed that higher cortical function deficits (HCFDs), including frontal network syndromes (FNS), were common in people after stroke. Both HCFDs and FNS were frequent, no matter where in the brain the stroke occurred [7–10]. An attempt was made to provide a multidisciplinary yet comprehensive bedside evaluation with the COCONUT tool [11]. This was found to be a valid and practical tool for both cognitive syndromes (CS) and emotional intelligence (EI) assessment in stroke patients. As both CS and FNS were noted to be frequent in stroke, subsequent FNS subtests and neuroimaging revealed that disinhibition, word list generation, a 5-word memory testing, and PET brain imaging may help distinguish the three most common dementia subtypes for example [12]. Furthermore, as neurological syndromes present from hyper-acute to acute, subacute, and chronic time frames, a hierarchical clinical assessment is proposed, depending on the clinical urgency and degree of cooperation by the patient. A stepwise, hierarchical approach largely determined by the level of consciousness and degree of cooperation is presented (Fig. 1.2).

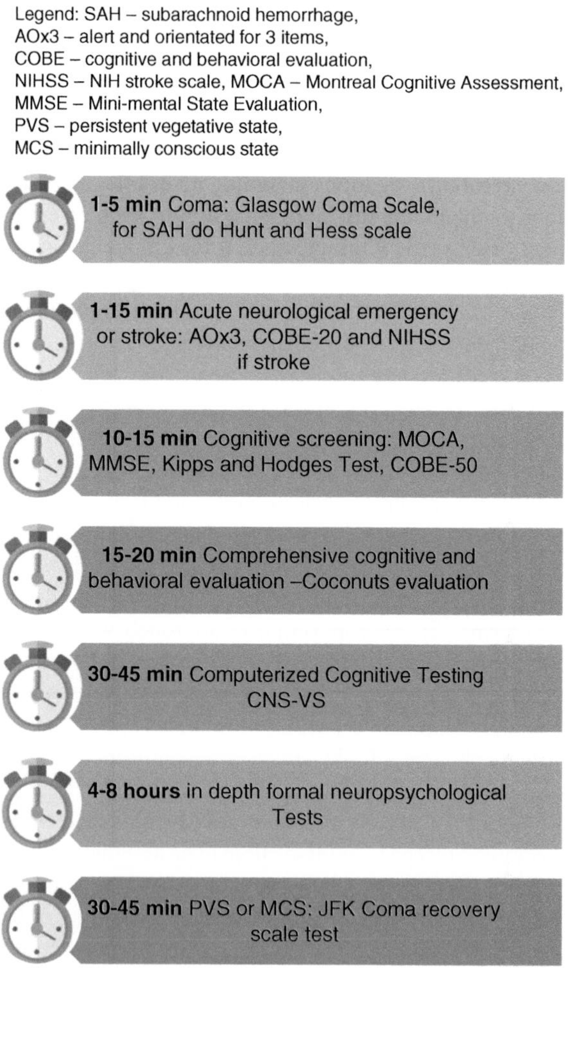

Fig. 1.2 Hierarchy of test choices according to time and neurological urgency. Legend: *SAH* subarachnoid hemorrhage, *AOx3* alert and orientated for 3 items, *COBE* cognitive and behavioral evaluation, *NIHSS* NIH stroke scale, *MOCA* Montreal cognitive assessment, *MMSE* mini-mental state evaluation, *PVS* persistent vegetative state, *MCS* minimally conscious state

Legend: SAH – subarachnoid hemorrhage,
AOx3 – alert and orientated for 3 items,
COBE – cognitive and behavioral evaluation,
NIHSS – NIH stroke scale, MOCA – Montreal Cognitive Assessment,
MMSE – Mini-mental State Evaluation,
PVS – persistent vegetative state,
MCS – minimally conscious state

1-5 min Coma: Glasgow Coma Scale, for SAH do Hunt and Hess scale

1-15 min Acute neurological emergency or stroke: AOx3, COBE-20 and NIHSS if stroke

10-15 min Cognitive screening: MOCA, MMSE, Kipps and Hodges Test, COBE-50

15-20 min Comprehensive cognitive and behavioral evaluation –Coconuts evaluation

30-45 min Computerized Cognitive Testing CNS-VS

4-8 hours in depth formal neuropsychological Tests

30-45 min PVS or MCS: JFK Coma recovery scale test

Cognitive Reserve May Mask Brain Pathology Until Late in Certain Brain Disease Processes

People with similar cognitive impairment may have markedly different Alzheimer's disease (AD) pathology for example, depending on their degree of brain reserve and cognitive reserve. Because of the cognitive reserve hypothesis, clinical examination alone cannot discern cognitive impairment. The cognitive reserve hypothesis proposes that people with similar cognitive impairments or even no impairment at all may nevertheless have rampant Alzheimer pathology. Hence, clinical psychometric testing is unlikely to reliably diagnose many people that may benefit from specific disease therapies. Metabolic testing with positron emission tomography (PET) brain scanning is known to improve diagnosis and extend the window of AD diagnosis into the mild clinical and even preclinical phase.

Cognitive and Behavioral Neurology Is Particularly Challenging: Thirty Three Stumbling Blocks of Cognitive and Behavioral Neurology

Devinksy opined in his excellent treatise on the subject, "Mental Status Exam 100 Maxims" that evaluation of mental status has an "undeservedly bad reputation and is systematic and hierarchical." He further lamented that "One only has to read a detailed and lengthy neuropsychological report or obsessive language examination to conclude that a busy clinician has no time fussing over higher cortical function assessment!" [13]. From my own perspective, the following challenges are most pertinent:

1. There may be no symptoms or signs and even denial of symptoms.
2. Positive heralding symptoms such as pain or hyperfunction are less common than negative symptoms such as aphasia, paralysis, or vision loss.
3. The doctor may get it wrong – we are prone to cognitive errors and errors of commission in diagnostic decision-making as well as technical examination errors. Groopman assembled more than a dozen types of errors that doctors make in patient evaluation including commission errors, confirmation bias, and the "Zebra Retreat" and avoiding contemplation of a rare diagnosis for example [14].
4. The patient may get it wrong – patients may not volunteer, underestimate, or even frankly deny the existence of a deficit or disease. Anosognosia, denial of disease, and anosodiaphoria are some of the more dramatic examples.
5. The brain may get it wrong – cognition fluctuates during the course of the day even in normal people. In the context of neurological disease, this may be even more profound, as occurs with progressive Lewy body disease for example.
6. Neurological lesions may be "silent" both to the patient and to the doctor. Examples include silent strokes depicted only by MRI imaging or only by PET

brain scanning in individuals with high cognitive reserve and incipient Alzheimer's dementia. "Whispering strokes" refer to presentations of stroke that are so mild that they are often ignored yet pose a risk for subsequent stroke [15].

7. Neurological syndromes may be present only when concomitant metabolic upset, infection, or medication leads to the "unmasking of deficits" such as a mild aphasia after a stroke syndrome that has either completely or almost completely recovered.

8. The hodological nature of brain deficits has both local and remote effects. Syndromes we normally attribute to one part of the brain, for example frontal lobe syndromes, may arise from the very posterior part of the brain or even brainstem and cerebellum. This observation underlies the complexity and pervasiveness of the frontal networks and diaschisis effects that influence all other brain regions

9. The primary syndrome may be due to a lesion that may allow the emergence of others. These have been referred to as "suppressed networks." An example would be the artistic ability after left hemisphere lesions due to stroke or dementia and imitation behavior due to frontal lobe lesions.

10. The cerebral pathophysiology may be due to electrical, chemical, or autoimmune perturbations. This impacts the type of imaging tools (MRI diffusion tensor imaging, EEG, PET brain imaging) that need to be deployed for facilitating a precise diagnosis. If not, the diagnosis may be missed altogether.

11. The presenting syndrome may be due to transient electrical phenomenon. Intermittent frontal lobe or temporal lobe epilepsy may be associated with a differing interictal presentation; for example, the "forced normalization" syndrome and other difficult diagnoses such as poriomania, gelastic epilepsy, ictal aphasia and proprioceptive reflex epilepsy, and ictal aphasia.

12. The clinical method has moved beyond anatomical lesion localization due to the complexity of brain networks.

13. The hub failure hypothesis posits that certain heteromodal association cortices are most prone to failure, no matter what the pathophysiological process demands. Hence, it may be more appropriate to think more in terms of networktopathies.

14. We have been too memory focused and attributing the cause to "early Alzheimer's disease" when in fact inattention, abulia, or fluctuating cognition may cause dysmemory.

15. We have been too neurological deficit focused as an increase in ability (artistry or musical) or activity (hemiballismus, mania) may be the presenting symptom.

16. We have been too pharmacocentric and underestimated neuroplasticity and relatively neglected powerful inherent therapies (music, art, meditation, device therapies).

17. Misdiagnosis remains rife with abulia and aprosodia diagnosed as depression and autoimmune encephalopathies misdiagnosed as psychiatric conditions.

18. Neurological syndromes may be present only when concomitant metabolic upset, infection, or medication leads to the unmasking of deficits such as a mild

aphasia after a stroke syndrome that has already completely or almost completely recovered.

19. Chemical aberrations may be the cause of a cognitive and behavioral impairment and may present as not only a more obvious syndrome such as Parkinson's but also more covert presentations with diagnostic difficulty as with the serotonin syndrome.

20. Frontotemporal degenerations and syndromes are frequently missed. Over one-third of patients offer no complaints or symptoms and neuropsychological testing itself is often normal or only mildly impaired.

21. Frontotemporal degenerations and syndromes may escape detection with the most common mental state screening tests, the MMSE, MOCA's being in the normal range. Even the Frontal Assessment Battery may be within normal range. Hence, they may miss the entry criteria for further neuropsychological and behavioral testing.

22. Frontotemporal degenerations and syndromes may be missed because the frequently co-occurring abulia may obviate neuropsychological and behavioral testing.

23. There is a long history of the cognitive–behavioral dissonance or normal neuropsychological tests with dramatically abnormal behavioral tests. This stems back to the 1848 Boston Crow Bar Case and Arnold Pick in his landmark description of FTD (Pick's disease) also noted presentation with inhibition and abulias, but not cognitive impairment as a rule.

24. The marked clinical cognitive-behavioral dissociation/sundering may further delay diagnosis because their language skills and cognitive skills are convincing.

25. Relying solely on anatomical neuroimaging with routine MRI may be unrevealing and often needs to include functional imaging such as with PET brain scanning.

26. State-dependent functions (aminergic neurotransmitters) include the frontal network system and ascending reticular activating system (ARAS) mediating rapid modulations of information processing. When intact, there is normal maintenance of mood, arousal, attention, and motivation. With no localizing value, deficiencies of state-dependent functions impact performance in all cognitive processes tasks and significantly affect the mental status examination.

27. Metabolic disorders, medication effects, multifocal lesions, and frontal lobe damage (impairment of top-down regulation) disrupt state-dependent mental functions.

28. Domains of cognitive processes are interactive, with an impairment in one influencing the performance in another.

29. No standardized tests exist for most behavioral syndromes such as simultanagnosia, agnosia, prosopagnosia, and the vast realm of human behavior including foresight, compassion, judgment, insight, curiosity, strength of will, and problem-solving ability.

30. The many so-called functional neurological disorders or hysterical presentations turn out to be "organic" illness.

31. The front (frontal lobes and their networks) and the back of the brain (visual network) contain the two most extensive brain networks. The majority of their syndromes need to be elicited by an assiduous history.
32. From an initial deficit (progressive aphasia of the frontal lobe type and non-fluent and semantic subtypes) may develop hyperfunction such as artistry. Both require neurological monitoring and management.
33. Normalcy, psychiatric, and neurological syndromes overlap.

Hyman has recommended that many of the categorically defined DSM disorders may be better described numerically and that in general, mental disorders should be viewed as dimensional traits (quantitative traits) in a continuity with the so-called "normal" state. Diagnostic classications, such as the DSM-V and ICD-10 have been regarded as atheoretical due to accumulating evidence that categorically distinct disease entities are not neurobiologically appropriate. Rather, there exist continua between the various syndromes, for example, schizophrenia and bipolar affective disorder and depression and anxiety disorders. The continua also exist between normalcy and psychosis. Currently, these are termed comorbid disorders. Genetic support from the polygenic mode of inheritance supports his premise as these characterize most mental impairment states. Specific examples include attention-deficit hyperactivity disorder, autism, depression, and schizophrenia. Unsurprisingly, a large proportion of clinical patients do not fit neatly into any DSM-V criteria with the consequence of being labeled with the rather uninformative "not otherwise specified" (NOS) all-encompassing category. Furthermore, a significant number of patients with DSM-V diagnoses qualify for more than one and sometimes multiple diagnoses. These are then conveniently termed called co-morbid disorders as occurs with entities such as bipolar disease, substance abuse, major depression and anxiety. The latter may well be different presentations of the same underlying gene at risk. It seems more likely or prudent to regard a particular pathophysiological process causing several different symptoms defined by the DSM-V. Comorbidity is more likely an artifact caused by the lumping and splitting of syndromes and symptoms. Further confirmation comes from the clinical findings that neuropharmacological agents do not adhere to the DSM-V boundaries of stipulated disorders. Hence, antidepressants treat anxiety, obsessive compulsive disorder, and depression, and antipsychotic drugs treat bipolar disorder, schizophrenia, Tourette's disorder, schizoaffective disorder, and Huntington's disease [16]. Increasingly, neuroimaging is coming to the rescue. Both metabolic PET brain scanning and MRI-based intrinsic connectivity scans have been for the first time used as biomarkers in severe depression. Metabolic PET scan reveals hypermetabolism in the subgenual cingulate cortex with normalization after successful antidepressant therapy [17]. The situation is urgent with depression affecting 300 million people globally by 2020 (WHO), and the second cause of disability and premature death is psychiatric disorder. Furthermore, psychological stress increases the risk for physical illness including cardiovascular and cerebrovascular disease. As has occurred with neurology and to some extent biological psychiatry, employing a neural circuit approach is advocated. Treating individual symptoms (working memory impairment hallucinations, anxiety) separately, by using dimensional approaches with quantitative scales, that are based on neuroscience, genetics and neuroimaging may be a more neurobiologically appropriate approach. From such an approach, a more expansive spectrum of disorders emerges (anxiety would include generalized anxiety disorders, post-traumatic stress disorders, social phobias). There is an urgent need to formulate diagnoses using clinical symptoms and signs as well as considering the pathophysiology of disorders. This was particularly well illustrated by the true story a young woman with a life-threatening autoimmune encephalitis that was repeatedly misdiagnosed with a number of psychiatric conditions chronicled in her New York Times bestseller book and accompanying movie "Brain on Fire." Only when a brain biopsy was performed with the correct diagnosis of autoimmune encephalitis made and subsequent intravenous immune globulin was curative [18].

A new paradigmatic approach has been evolving – the human connectomic analysis for evaluating management of higher cortical function. This has strong evolutionary foundations that relate well to pathophysiological and neuroimaging points of view. Sebastian Seung, in his book *Connectome*, used a good example: "Studying mental disorders without connectomics is like researching infectious diseases without a microscope. Changing our brains is all about changing our connectome" [19]. The concept connectomics is a major landmark in human history and we are at a crossroad with opportunities to impact treatment approaches. Hence, Chap. 2 follows with an overview of our current understanding of human connectomics.

References

1. Crossley MA, Scott J, et al. The hubs of the human connectome are generally implicated in the anatomy of brain disorders. Brain. 2014;137:2382–95.
2. Boustani M, Peterson B, Hanson L, et al. Screening for dementia in primary care: a summary of the evidence for the US preventive services task force. Ann Intern Med. 2003;138:927–37.
3. Bredesen D. The end of Alzheimer's: the first program to prevent and reverse cognitive decline. New York: Penguin Random House; 2017.
4. AcAtee CP. Fitness, nutrition and the molecular basis of chronic disease. Biotechnol Genet Eng Rev. 2013;29:1–23.
5. Pasinettu GM, Eberstein JA. Metabolic syndrome and the role of dietary lifestyles in Alzheimer's disease. J Neurochem. 2008;106(4):1503–14.
6. Saver JL. Comments, opinions and reviews. Time Is Brain—Quantified Stroke. 2006;37:263–6.
7. Hoffmann M, Sacco RS, Mohr JP, Tatemichi TK. Higher cortical function deficits among acute stroke patients: the stroke data Bank experience. J Stroke Cerebrovasc Dis. 1997;6:114–20.
8. Hoffmann M. Higher cortical function deficits after stroke. An analysis of 1000 patients from a dedicated cognitive stroke registry. Neurorehabil Neural Repair. 2001;15:113–27.
9. Hoffmann M, Schmitt F. Metacognition in stroke: bedside assessment and relation to location, size, and stroke severity. Cogn Behav Neurol. 2006;19(2):85–94.
10. Hoffmann M, Schmitt F. Cognitive impairment in isolated subtentorial stroke. Acta Neuol Scand. 2004;109:14–24.
11. Hoffmann M, Schmitt F, Bromley E. Comprehensive cognitive neurological assessment in stroke. Acta Neurol Scand. 2009;119(3):162–71.

12. Hoffmann M. Frontal network syndrome testing: clinical tests and positron emission tomography brain imaging help distinguish the 3 most common dementia subtypes. Am J Alzheimers Dis Other Dement. 2103;28:477–84.
13. Devinsky O. Behavioral neurology 100 maxims. London: E. Arnold; 1992.
14. Groopman J. How doctors think. New York: Mariner Books; 2008.
15. Windham BG, et al. Covert neurological symptoms associated with silent infarcts from midlife to older age. The atherosclerosis risk in communities study. Stroke. 2012;43:1218–23.
16. Hyman SE. Can neuroscience be integrated into the DSM-V? Nat Rev Neurosci. 2007;8:725–32.
17. Mayberg HS, Brannan SK, Jerabek PA, et al. Cingulate function in depression: a potential predictor of treatment response. Neuroreport. 1997;8:1057–61.
18. Cahalan S. Brain on fire: my month of madness. New York: Simon and Schuster; 2012.
19. Seung S. Connectome. How the Brain's wiring makes us who we are. New York: Houghton, Mifflin, Harcourt Publishing Company; 2012.

Chapter 2
Neuroanatomical and Neurophysiological Underpinnings of Cognition and Behavior: Cerebral Networks and Intrinsic Brain Networks

For almost a century, Brodmann's 52 component cytoarchitectural brain map has served clinical neuroscience, neurology, and psychology in the topographical appreciation of differing brain regions (Fig. 2.1) [1]. Subsequent neurosurgical needs resulted in the immensely popular Talairach Tournoux brain atlas for three-dimensional coordinates of brain regions and components [2]. From a purely clinical point of view, Mesulam's clinical large-scale network approach has long been popular in understanding higher cortical function deficit presentations [3]. He conceived of the 5 channel-dependent networks and the 5 frontal subcortical networks proposed by Cummings and Lichter represent complementary understanding of the more intricate frontal subsystems [4]. The neurotransmitter-based state or chemical projections are yet another facet to the intricacies of brain networks (Table 2.1). With the human cerebral cortex comprising 20 billion neurons over 2.5 meter squared, primary motor, sensory, visual, and auditory regions only constitute ~10%, with the remainder being secondary and tertiary association cortices. The latter are the neurobiological substrates of higher cortical functions. More recently, using an array of neuroimaging techniques (myelin, fMRI, connectivity, task maps), the human brain map has been redefined from 52 Brodmann areas to 360 areas (Fig. 2.2) [5].

These mesoscale and microscopic scale network systems have served us well for the past few decades. With refinements of our technological abilities (functional MRI based) in deciphering complex networks, aided in no small way by mathematical network science, a new era of complex brain network systems has emerged, the mesoscale networks termed intrinsic connectivity networks (ICNs).

© Springer Nature Switzerland AG 2020
M. Hoffmann, *Clinical Mentation Evaluation*,
https://doi.org/10.1007/978-3-030-46324-3_2

Fig. 2.1 Brodmann areas, primary areas, and unimodal and tertiary association areas. Red and blue areas depict primary motor and primary sensory areas such as tactile, visual, and auditory. Orange depicts supplementary motor areas and pale blue unimodal association areas. The white regions depict higher order, heteromodal association areas or tertiary association areas. Legend: *RF* rolandic fissure. (Figure credit with permission from: Fuster [15])

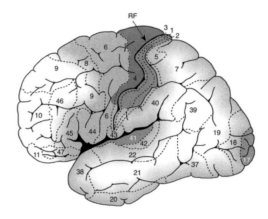

Table 2.1 The five channel dependent networks, five frontal subcortical networks and the principal neurotransmitter based networks

A. Channel-dependent networks
1. Left dominant, peri-sylvian network for language
2. Right dominant, dorsal frontoparietal network for spatial orientation
3. Occipitotemporal, ventral network for face and object recognition
4. Limbic network for explicit episodic memory and emotion
5. Prefrontal network for executive control of cognition and comportment
B. Frontal subcortical circuits (channel dependent)
1. Dorsolateral
2. Orbitofrontal
3. Anterior cingulate
4. Oculomotor
5. Motor
C. Principal chemical projections to the cerebral cortex (state-dependent systems)
1. Cholinergic projections from the nucleus basalis of Meynert
2. Histaminergic projections from the hypothalamus
3. Dopaminergic projections from the ventral tegmental area
4. Serotonergic projections from brainstem raphe nuclei
5. Noradrenergic projections from the locus ceruleus
6. Orexin projections from hypothalamus

Large-Scale Brain Networks

Large-scale intrinsic networks subserve human brain function, reflecting a temporal activation coupling of widely distributed and disparate cerebral regions. Their metabolic demands also consume the majority of the brain's energy budget. ICN analysis has been very insightful both in diagnosis and in being able to

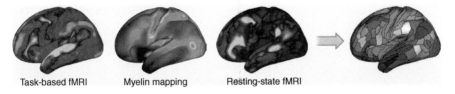

Task-based fMRI   Myelin mapping   Resting-state fMRI

Fig. 2.2 Brain map redefined from 52 Brodmann areas to 360, using myelin, fMRI, connectivity, task maps [5]

understand the pathophysiology of many complex neurological and neuropsychiatric disorders such as Alzheimer's disease (AD) and depression. For example, the "march" of neurodegenerative disease such as tau and amyloid deposits in AD that maps very closely to the default mode network (DMN) and the salience network that corresponds to frontotemporal disorders (FTD) are both good examples of ICN contributions to the pathophysiological understanding of these conditions. Furthermore, with respect to mild cognitive impairment (MCI), network signatures are considered the most sensitive and also the earliest "biomarkers" of these conditions. To date, functional connectivity of the DMN has been implicated in many other conditions in addition to AD and include depression, autism, schizophrenia, depression, epilepsy, and amyotrophic lateral sclerosis. This has also substantiated the growing trend for dimensional approaches in psychiatric conditions as opposed to categorical entities [6].

During the past two decades, several major ICNs have been identified and the number is growing.

Yeo, Buckner, and Krienen identified a 7-network parcellation of the human cortex as well as a 17 parcellation network with fractionation of the 7-network parcellation into smaller networks (Fig. 2.3) [7] (Tables 2.2 and 2.3).

The Neurobiology and Principles of Connectivity
(Figs. 2.4 and 2.5) [6, 9, 10]

1. Both spatially compact or clustered communities (provincial hubs) and long-range connections characterize brain networks.
2. Brain networks are characterized by features of both global communication and functional integration, both metabolically costly.
3. The long-range connections enable efficient neural communication between remote brain regions as functionally distinct regions.
4. Central hub regions are features of most long-range connections with diverse connections encompassing a wide range of functions.

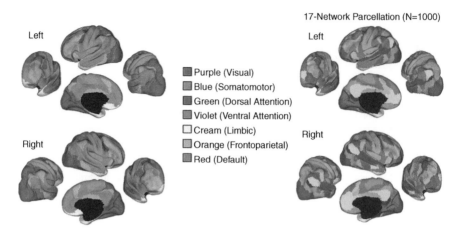

Fig. 2.3 Buckners 7 and 17 intrinsic functional connectivity brain networks [7]

Table 2.2 Current number of described ICNs that are clinically relevant [8]

1. Default mode network (mentalizing)
2. Salience (ventral attention)
3. Dorsal attention
4. Executive control
5. Limbic
6. Language
7. Sensorimotor
8. Motor
9. Visual
10. Mirroring network
11. Limbic mirroring network

5. The central hub regions also connect extensively to each other so that they comprises a central core of "rich clubs" within brain networks.
6. They subserve higher cortical functions by means of synchronized oscillations and the co-activations of a number of distributed brain regions.
7. There is accruing evidence of abnormal connectivity in many neurological and neuropsychiatric disorders.
8. Important clinical implications are that ICN analysis can detect distinct patterns of network disruption in severe neurodegenerative diseases (NDD) including depression. Even more important is that these network abnormalities may depict intermediate clinical phenotypes that will allow earlier detection where brain pathology exists but not yet clinical syndromes [11].
9. Various cerebral disorders associated with metabolic impairment, such as the metabolic syndrome, present with network abnormalities in selectively in both

Table 2.3 Components of the better known cognitive networks

Salience network components/nodes
1. Anterior insula
2. Dorsal anterior cingulate
3. Superior temporal pole
4. DLPFC (46)
5. SMA and pre-SMA
6. Operculum (frontal, temporal, parietal components)
7. Subcortical (amygdala, striato-pallidum, DM thalamus, hypothalamus, PAG, SN, VTA)
Executive control network, right DLPFC components/nodes
1. Bilateral DLPFC
2. Ventrolateral PFC
3. Dorsomedial PFC
4. Lateral parietal
5. Left fronto-insula
6. Coupled with caudate, anterior thalamus
DMN components/nodes
1. Medial parietal area
2. Medial prefrontal area
3. Lateral parietal area
4. Lateral temporal cortex

DLPFC dorsolateral prefrontal cortex; *SMA* supplementary motor area; *PAG* peri acqueductal gray matter; *SN* substantia nigra; *VTA* ventral tegmental area; *PFC* prefrontal cortex; *DM* dorsomedial

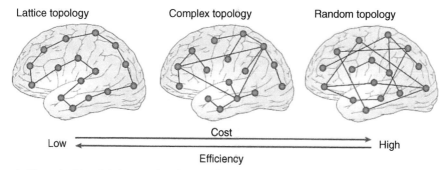

- Lattice: wired to minimize cost but does not favor global integration of information processing
- Random: incurs a high wiring cost due to large number of long distance connections, where each node is connected on average to two other nodes. Brain integrative processing is maximized by random topology
- Human brain networks are between these two extremes. Both clusters of lattice like short distance connections and long distance high cost components between connector hubs

Fig. 2.4 The economy of brain network organization. Bullmore [16]

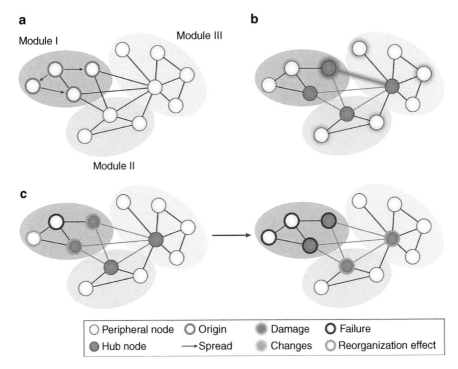

Fig. 2.5 Cascading network failure. The connectome consists of modules (**a**) and this arrangement shapes the way disease spreads, as illustrated by damaged hub nodes (red) and their associated connections (red) in (**b**). The initial failure in one node cascades to others. However, a failing network node may also trigger compensatory consequences in nodes adjacent to the damaged node, which then assumes the role played by the damaged nodes (green) in efforts to sustain brain function (**c**) [12]

the high cost hub components as well as the long-distance connections. Such highly connected regions, termed "hot spots," are particularly vulnerable and occur in many disease processes because of their centrality in the network. What follows is that they become inordinately disruptive to entire global networks.

10. Alzheimer's disease (AD) selectively impacts the most expensive hub nodes of a brain network. One of the findings is a reduction in degree of long-distance connections, with reduced network efficiency and increased clustering. This network reconfiguration may be viewed as a cost-efficiency trade-off by lowering metabolic connections costs but with the loss of integrative capacity.

11. The vulnerability of high-cost hubs have been attributed to extensive dendritic branching, increased synaptic density of pyramidal neurons, as well as profound metabolic demands.

12. Such findings are not restricted to AD but also to many other neurological diseases. Brain regions with high value hubs by fMRI networks, notably the medial posterior parietal cortex, are usually the first to be impacted by beta amyloid deposition.

13. In multiple sclerosis, the impact is also primarily on the most expensive (longest) connections in the network.
14. In general, neurodegenerative diseases begin with a primary epicenter, where after spreading occurs along the connectivity relating to these epicenters. The more local modular networks are first implicated and are termed the "ignition point" of neurodegenerative disorders. The cascading network failure theory as it pertains to AD has the initial failure within the default mode network hubs.
15. A so-called cascading network failure occurs with the spreading of disease involving more and more of the network nodes [12].
16. Cross disorder connectomics is a concept proposed by Van den Heuvel and Sporns, whereby brain disorders are conceived of as dysfunction of neural networks that extend across conventional network as well as known diagnostic boundaries. Hence, a "connectotyping" is a connectivity spanning multiple brain conditions. Cross disorder connectomics enables our understanding of disease comorbidities we so often encounter particular in psychiatric conditions [12]
17. Another facet to cross-disorder connectomics would be determining on how connectome alterations might preempt behavioral changes, such as with mild cognitive impairment.
18. Cross-disorder connectotyping has the potential of becoming a precision medicine tool. Precision connectomics may potentially be capable of producing dimensional maps of an individual's particular connectivity profile. This in turn might relate to the individual's propensity to brain disorders as well as vulnerability and resilience to such conditions [12].
19. Perhaps most noteworthy is the study by Crossley et al. proposing from the data that high-cost/high-value hubs of the human brain networks are more likely to be anatomically abnormal than non-hubs in many (if not all) brain disorders [13].

Brain Networks and the Hodological Perspective

The diaschisis phenomenon helps explain that syndromes may be due to remote hypoactivation after a brain lesion. Importantly, the temporal reorganization of the connectome that is remote to the causative lesion may be representative of a kind of surrogate marker of recovery. It is well known that network dysfunction may at times, also extend into the opposite intact hemisphere as can be seen with certain aphasias. Several different forms of diaschisis have been proposed by Carrera and Tononi [14] (Fig. 2.6).

- *Diaschisis at rest*: A hypometabolism distant to the lesion without stimulation or activation.
- *Functional diaschisis*: Alteration of responsiveness of a neural network remote from a lesion with physiological activation such as moving a hand and only causing cerebellar deactivation secondary to basal ganglia lesion.
- *Connectional diaschisis*: After circumscribed lesions, widespread remote connectivity changes may occur in both hemispheres. For example, a decrease in

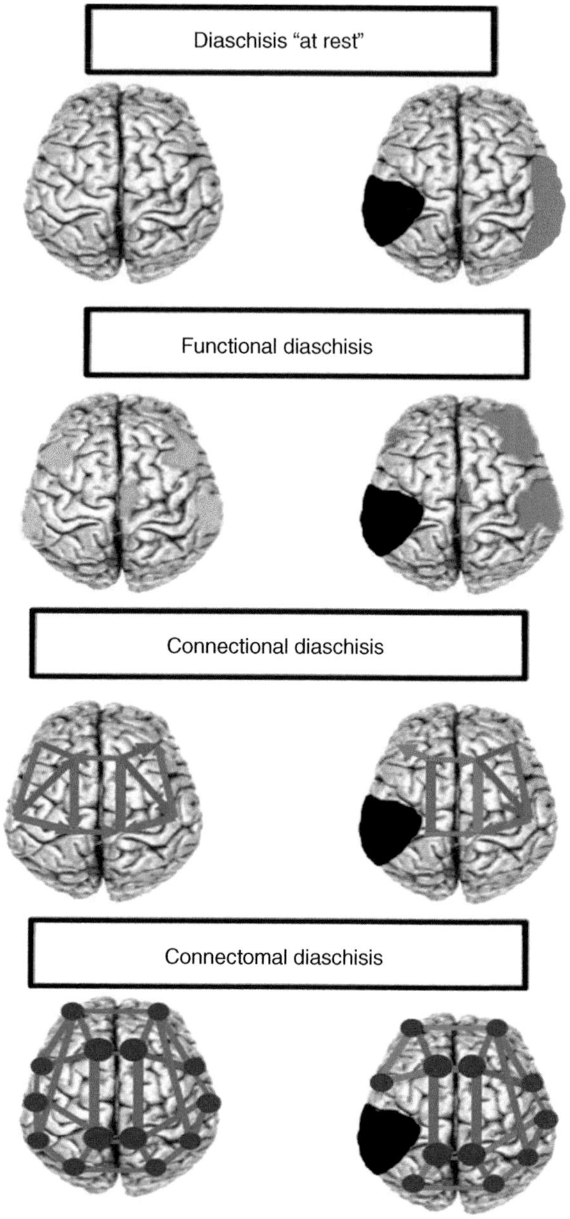

Fig. 2.6 A connectomal
perspective: clinical [14]

interhemisphere connectivity of both motor networks has been documented after
isolated subcortical strokes.

- *Connectomal diaschisis*: Contemporary neuroimaging tools including diffusion tensor imaging (DTI), fMRI, MEG, and high-density EEG (HdEEG) have
  the highest temporal resolution (so less spatial resolution) and can measure

functional coupling between brain areas. The most pronounced impacts on the connectome occur with the cortical midline lesions, the temporo-parietal junction (BA 5 and 7), and the frontal regions (BA 46 and 8).

Remote effects from diaschisis may also refer to increased function or abilities. These include newly found artistry with left frontal or left temporal lobe lesion, the acquired Savant syndrome, and other examples such as hyper-connectivity syndromes due to post-traumatic stress syndrome (PTSD) and Klüver–Bucy syndrome. People with PTSD may at times relive previously stressful experiences associated with "flashbacks". These comprise of multi-sensory experiences associated with powerful emotional features such as anger outbursts as well as hypervigilance, visual hallucinations, vivid memories, nightmares, visual hallucinations, hyper-arousal and exaggerated startle responses. This syndrome may be regarded as an occipito-amygdaloid disconnection syndrome.

References

1. Brodmann K. Vergleichende Lokalisationslehre der Großhirnrinde in ihren Prinzipien dargestellt auf Grund des Zellenbaues. Barth, Leipzig, 1909. English translation: Garey LJ. Brodmann's localization in the cerebral cortex. London: Smith Gordon; 1994.
2. Talairach J, Tournoux P. Co-planar stereotaxic atlas of the human brain. New York: Thieme Medical Publishers Inc, 1988.
3. Mesulam M-M. Large scale neurocognitive networks and distributed processing for attention, language and memory. Ann Neurol. 1990;28:597–613.
4. Chow TW, Cummings JL. Frontal subcortical circuits. In: Miller B, Cummings JL, editors. The human frontal lobes. New York: The Guilford Press; 2009.
5. Thomas Yeo BT, Eickhoff SB. A modern map of the human cerebral cortex. Nature. 2016;536:152–4. Glasser MF, Coalson TS, Robinson EC et al. Nature 2016;536:171–178
6. Buckner RL, Krienen FM. The evolution of distributed association networks in the human brain. Trends Cogn Sci. 2013;17:648–65.
7. Yeo BTT, Krienen FM, Sepulcre J, Buckner RL, et al. The organization of the human cerebral cortex estimated by intrinsic functional connectivity. J Neurophysiol. 2011;106:1125–65.
8. Barrett LF, Satpute AB. Large scale brain networks in affective and social neuroscience: towards an integrative functional architecture of the brain. Curr Opin Neurobiol. 2013;23:361–72.
9. Kaiser M, Varier S. Evolution and development of brain networks from Caenorhabditis elegans to Homo sapiens. Network. 2011;22:143–7.
10. Zhu DJ, et al. Connectome scale assessments of structural and functional connectivity in MCI. Hum Brain Mapp. 2014;35:2911–23.
11. Zeng LL, Shen H, Liu L, et al. Identifying major depression using whole brain functional connectivity: a multivariate pattern analysis. Brain. 2012;135:1498–507.
12. Van den Heuvel MP, Sporns O. A cross disorder connectome landscape of brain dysconnectivity. Nat Rev Neurosci. 2019;20:435–46.
13. Crossley N, Mechelli A, Scott J, et al. The hubs of the human connectome are generally implicated in the anatomy of brain disorders. Brain. 2014;137:2382–95.
14. Carrera E, Tononi G. Diaschisis: past, present and future. Brain. 2014;137:2408–22.
15. Fuster JM. The Prefrontal Cortex. 4th ed. Amsterdam: Elsevier; 2008.
16. Bullmore E, Sporns O. The economy of brain network organization and adjust reference to read; Bullmore E, Sporns O. The economy of brain network organization. Nature Neuroscience Reviews 2012;13:336–49.

Chapter 3
How Do Patients Present? Acute and Chronic Presentations

Certain stereotyped neurological presentations are typical in the clinic, hospital, or emergency room environment (Table 3.1).

Stroke Presentations

Stroke mostly presents with elementary neurological syndromes associated with positive imaging by multimodality MRI scanning. The most commonly employed stroke assessment scale, the NIHSS, is used for both emergently assessing degree of deficit and guiding thrombolytic therapy. Usually the challenge is with diagnosing the clinical syndrome, given the lesion seen on brain scanning.

Table 3.1 Acute and chronic presentations of cognitive and behavioral disorders

A. Acute presentations
Stroke
Altered mental status and delirium
Encephalopathies
Seizures
B. Chronic presentation including mild cognitive impairment (MCI), mild behavioral impairment (MBI), and dementia presentations
MCI spectrum presentation (subjective to moderate MCI to incipient dementia)
MBI
Dementias
Elementary neurological symptoms such as tremor as first sign of ND disease
Unusual, unexplained symptoms – hysteria, somatic disorder

ND neurodegenerative disease

© Springer Nature Switzerland AG 2020
M. Hoffmann, *Clinical Mentation Evaluation*,
https://doi.org/10.1007/978-3-030-46324-3_3

Altered Mental Status and the Delirium Spectrum of Disorders

In many tertiary centers, the most common consultation of all, is for the cause of altered mental status. Patients with delirium patients may be agitated, which is appropriately termed hyperactive delirium, and has a frequency of about 25% of altered mental status cases. The etiology is of paramount importance and includes a formidable list of entities that require expedited consideration. A comprehensive yet easily memorized pneumonic is that of Maracantonio:

D-e-l-i-r-i-u-m etiology

Drugs, **e**lectrolyte disturbance, **l**ack of drugs, **i**nfections, **r**educed sensory input, **i**ntracranial lesions (infection, stroke, hemorrhage, tumor) **u**rinary sepsis (cystocerebral syndrome) **m**yocardial and pulmonary [1].

Encephalopathies

These encompass an extensive differential spanning not only the brain diseases but also all organ systems. Many encephalopathic syndromes may have covert presentations, such as occurs with certain chronic medical disorders with minimal hepatic encephalopathy (MHE) being a good example. Hepatic encephalopathy is a neuropsychiatric and cognitive complication of chronic liver disease. Symptoms of MHE may be particularly subtle (inattention, executive dysfunction) or overt (coma, confusion, disorientation, ataxia), which are commonly evaluated by the West Haven Criteria with scores ranging from 0 to 4 (0 normal, 4 coma) and grades 1 and 2 in the MHE range. Pathologic mechanisms are related to elevated levels of ammonia, inflammation, low-grade cerebral edema, and neurotransmitter perturbations. The diagnosis of MHE requires psychometric and neurophysiological testing and at times magnetic resonance spectroscopic (MRS) measurement with the measurement of a specific calculation by MRS called "Hunters triangle" of diagnostic reliability. Herpes simplex encephalitis is another syndrome that may evade diagnosis, as particularly unusual and subtle cognitive and behavioral presentations are typical. The process may be fulminant with demise within days if not contemplated.

Seizures

Seizures are usually easily diagnosed clinically or by electroencephalography, but the entity of frontal lobe seizures almost always causes diagnostic confusion and difficulty and not infrequently a functional diagnosis or non-epileptic disorder diagnoses are made. Furthermore, most idiopathic generalized seizures are considered

Table 3.2 Clincal feature of frontal lobe seizures, frontal lobe seizure classification and other seizures that have behavioral syndromes

Clinical features of frontal lobe seizures
1. Auras
2. Vocalizations
3. Prominent motor manifestations
4. Brief duration
5. Clustering
6. Occurrence during sleep
Classification of FLE
1. Primary motor cortex seizures
2. Supplementary motor seizures
3. Cingulate seizures
4. Frontopolar seizures
5. Orbitofrontal complex focal motor seizures
6. Dorsolateral premotor seizures
7. Opercular seizures
Other seizure manifestations and syndromes occurring with epilepsy that may present with behavioral sequelae
1. Poriomania or wandering aimlessly
2. Procursive epilepsy or running epilepsy
3. Volvular epilepsy or waking repetitively in small circles
4. Ictal aphasia
5. Gelastic epilepsy
6. Transient epileptic amnesia
7. Autoscopy experiences
8. Déjà vu and jamais vu experiences
9. Forced normalization and the Gastaut-Geschwind syndrome
10. Reflex epilepsy: evocative stimuli due to visual (flickering light or red colors), auditory-induced startling, somatosensory, writing or reading induced, eating induced

likely to originate in the frontal lobes. Frontal lobe seizures, psychogenic non-epileptic seizures (PNES), the entity of nocturnal frontal lobe epilepsy (NFLE) and parasomnias and their differentiation, continue to perplex clinicians. NFLE and parasomnias have been shown to disinhibit central pattern generators albeit different mechanisms, resulting in similar manifestations of behaviors including the following (Table 3.2):

- Locomotion activity
- Bicycling activity
- Swimming activity
- Running activity
- NFLE and parasomnias coexist in ~30% of patients
- Approximately 90% of FLE originate during sleep

Table 3.3 MCI guidelines 2018

1. Assess for MCI with validated tools in appropriate scenarios.
2. Evaluate patients with MCI for modifiable risk factors.
3. Assess for functional impairment.
4. Assess for and treat behavioral/neuropsychiatric symptoms.
5. Monitor cognitive status of MCI over time.
6. Cognitively impairing medications should be discontinued wherever possible.
7. Clinicians may choose not to offer cholinesterase inhibitors (level B), and if offering, first discuss lack of evidence (level A).
8. Clinicians should recommend regular exercise (level B).
9. Clinicians may recommend cognitive training (level C).

The Challenge of Subjective Cognitive Impairment (SCI), Mild Cognitive Impairment (MCI), Mild Behavioral Impairment (MBI)

Mental status abnormalities are present in most, if not all, neurological disorders (vulnerable hub hypothesis) with 50–75% of people with MCI not diagnosed, yet some may be reversible. In addition, MCI diagnosis has inherent high false-positive and false-negative rates [2]. The neurodegenerative syndromes have a wide range of presentations from purely subjective reports (Richard Wetherill case: https://www.newscientist.com/article/mg18825301-300-how-brainpower-can-help-you-cheat-old-age/) to advanced dementia. It has been known for a long time that vascular disease comes first and underlies all of the major dementia groups.

The most recent MCI guidelines for assessment and management was published by Petersen et al. in 2018. These guidelines differed markedly from the memory-centric and pharmacocentric approach that characterized the past few decades [3]. A summarized version is presented in Table 3.3.

The Importance of the Underlying Vascular Basis of MCI and Dementias

There is a commonality of risk factors of stroke and dementia. Ten risk factors are associated with approximately 90% of strokes and over 90% of the stroke risk factors for stroke also pertain to dementias (Fig. 3.1). The only risk factors that differ for the dementias, include the presence of the APOE4 allele and a history of traumatic brain injury [4]. Stroke and dementia are now considered to be two extremes of vascular cognitive disorders in general and there exists a continuum (Fig. 3.2) from pure stroke to pure dementia, with most people lying somewhere in between the two entities [5]. The pathophysiology of the vascular contributions to the dementias may be briefly summarized as follows;

Fig. 3.1 The underlying vascular basis of MCI and dementia: commonality of risk factors. Ten risk factors associated with 90% of risk of stroke [4]	Stroke Risk Factors	(OR)	Alzheimer's Disease Risk Factors
	• Hypertension	(2.64)	• Hypertension
	• Cardiac causes	(2.38)	• Cardiac causes
	• Smoking current	(2.09)	• Diabetes
	• Apolipoprotein B/A1	(1.89)	• Smoking
	• Waist to hip ratio	(1.65)	• Alcohol excess
	• Alcohol intake	(1.51)	• Hypercholesterolemia
	• Diabetes Mellitus	(1.36)	• Hyperhomocysteinemia
	• Diet risk score	(1.35)	• Psychological stress
	• Depression	(1.35)	• Head injury
	• Psychosocial stress	(1.30)	• Apo E- 4 genotype
	• Physical exercise	(0.69)	

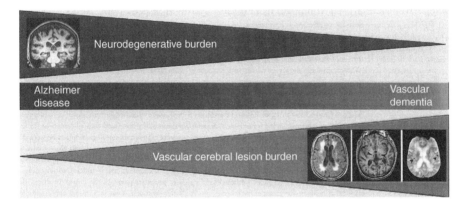

Fig. 3.2 The Vascular–dementia continuum [5]

- Vascular dysregulation in Alzheimer's has been known since ~1900 in contradistinction to the amyloid hypothesis.
- Age-dependent blood-brain barrier (BBB) permeability breakdown correlates with cognitive dysfunction.
- With BBB breakdown, misfolded protein deposition follows and subsequent toxicity of the protein.
- Beta-amyloid impairs mitochondrial function including increased production of reactive oxygen species with ultimate failure in cellular energy.
- The ensuing hypometabolism and toxicity cause both neuron and glial cell death and thereafter cerebral atrophy and cognition failure [6].

White matter hyperintensities (leukoaraiosis) are frequently noted by MRI scanning in both MH clinically normal, non-demented older adults and in those with established small vessel cerebrovascular disease. For many decades, both radiology and neurology dismissed these as incidental findings with little bearing of brain function. However, more recently, there is an awareness that clinically silent leukoaraiosis impacts cognitive aging with disproportionate effects on the frontal lobes. Leukoaraiosis

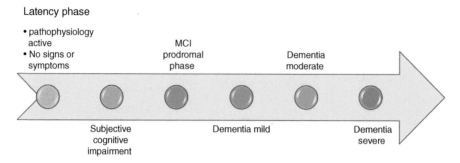

Fig. 3.3 Dementias are clinically and pathologically heterogeneous

is also strongly linked to small vessel cerebrovascular disease, and with its subcortical and periventricular predominance, frontal lobe dysfunction is evident. Neuroimaging by PET brain scanning with Pittsburgh compound B has documented that 20–30% of older adults that were clinically normal nevertheless were amyloid positive and had significant amyloid deposition in frontal and parietal brain regions. The amyloid may also cause increased frontoparietal activity on certain cognitive tasks accompanied by decreased activity of the right inferior prefrontal cortex. Phylogenetically, newer regions such as the frontal and temporal lobes are more susceptible to decline with aging. The frontal lobes in particular, seem preferentially vulnerable to decline. The cause of the propensity to decline process has been ascribed to changes in distributed networks as opposed to focal abnormalities. Aging is associated with many network changes and pathological processes which may not manifest clinically and frequently overlooked, and a rich cognitive diversity may be appreciated in the older population. Importantly, frontal lobe aging may be a malleable process through lifestyle and vascular risk factor management with both impeding cognitive decline and minimizing pathology. In addition, there is evidence that mixed pathologies underlie brain aging and these account for the majority of cases of dementia as determined by autopsy studies. This includes so called "normal" aging [7].

Dementia Presentations (Fig. 3.3)

The progressive decline begins "silently" in most cases and progresses over years and decades in the following manner:

- Latency phase: no signs or symptoms but already pathophysiological
- Subjective cognitive impairment
- MCI prodromal phase

    - Mild
    - Moderate
    - Severe

- Dementia

    - Mild
    - Moderate
    - Severe

- Behavioral impairment

    - Mild
    - Moderate
    - Severe

- Activities of daily living (basic)

    - Grooming, bathing, hygiene, eating, dressing, transferring

- Activities of daily living (instrumental)

    - Managing finances, driving, preparing meals, using devices, shopping

Dementias are clinically and pathologically heterogeneous with multiple subtypes now appreciated (Fig. 3.4). Another facet of complexity concerns the increasing number of classic dementia presentations being encountered that are treatable and even reversed [8]. Most of these can be identified by the proposed cognitive and behavioral evaluations. Perhaps the most striking example is the panoply of autoimmune encephalitis which manifests with florid behavioral neurological and neuropsychiatric syndromes that are frequently misdiagnosed or attributed to conversion disorders. The consequences of incorrect diagnosis of these syndromes are devastating, yet most can be significantly improved and many cured with immunosuppressive therapy such as IVIG and rituximab. These dramatic conditions have only recently been appreciated (Table 3.4).

Brain lesions and syndromes may present with a combination of cognitive, behavioral, and elementary neurological signs as well as seizures, neuropsychiatric, cerebrovascular, and general medical components. The cognitive and/or behavioral neurological impairment may be traced to each of these entities or at times a combination of them. Hence it is important that after the history, physical examination and investigative data are available, a composite evaluation is presented in the report. For example, in a young patient with mild traumatic brain injury post-IED blast exposure, the following assessment is typical:

1. Cognitive and behavioral: episodic dysmemory, executive dysfunction, abulia and disinhibition
2. Elementary neurological: anosmia, cervical radiculopathy, partial seizures, migraines
3. Neuropsychiatric: depression, anxiety, Post traumatic stress disorder (PTSD)
4. Cerebrovascular: hypertension, elevated body mass index, sleep apnea
5. General medical including drugs: many drugs are anticholinergic (~600), statins, hypotension

Pathophysiology: Post-traumatic brain injury syndrome with sequelae of cognitive, behavioral impairment, complicated by migraines and partial seizures.

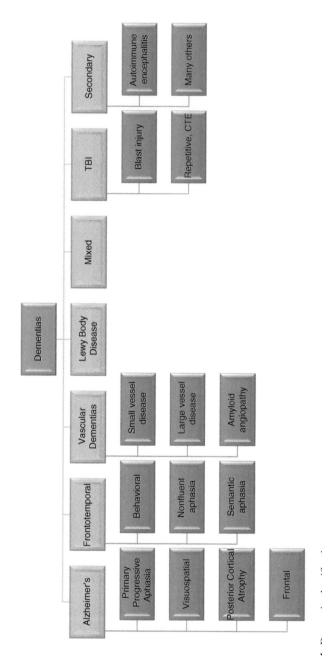

Fig. 3.4 Dementia classification

Table 3.4 Elementary neurological symptoms as first sign of neurodegenerative disease	*Motor systems*
	Tremor – first sign of neurodegenerative condition
	Bradykinesia, rigidity, gait impairment, resting tremor
	Chorea – Huntington's disease
	Cranial nerve related
	Anosmia – dementia, TBI, frontal lobe mass
	Eye movements
	Gaze palsy, – Wernicke's encephalopathy, progressive supranuclear palsy
	Visual hallucinations – Charles Bonnet, Lewy body disease, delirium
	Kayser Fleischer rings – Wilson' disease
	Gait
	Ataxia – leukoaraiosis, leukodystrophy, stroke, multiple sclerosis
	Neuromuscular
	Myoclonus – prionopathies, Alzheimer's disease, encephalopathy
	Neuropathy
	Muscle disease, wasting, fasciculations – Motor neuron disease and the frontotemporal dementia spectrum
	Dystonia – Wilson's disease, corticobasal disorder, Huntington's disease
	Cortical
	Frontal – field-dependent behavior
	Frontal lobe release signs – pouting, sucking and palmo-mental reflexes
	Alien limb – corticobasal disorder

With the diagnosis of cognitive and behavioral impairments, assessment of basic activities of daily living (ADL)'s with the help of an informant is required. Failure to be able to perform basic ADL's is a requirement for the diagnosis of dementia.

Unusual and Unexplained Symptoms

Misdiagnosis of hysteria with concomitant organic illness is considerable and there is a long history of previous hysterical diagnoses that are nowadays clearly organic neurological illnesses [9]. These syndromes are commonly encountered with varying incidence ranging from 4 to 12 per 100,000 per year [9, 10]. It has been estimated that approximately 30% of neurological outpatients have unexplained or marginally explained symptoms, at least by our currently known neurological disease categories [11]. In the subgroup of psychogenic non-epileptic seizure (PNES),

Table 3.5 Hysteria diagnosis mimics	
	Phantom limb pain
	Sensory trick in dystonia
	Various tremors
	Myasthenia gravis
	Dystonias, especially task specific; writer's cramp and musician's dystonia
	Epilepsia partialis continua
	Frontal lobe seizures
	Pure word deafness
	Alexia without agraphia
	Simultanagnosia
	Anosognosia
	Anton's syndrome

abnormalities in terms of MRI brain or EEG testing were found in 22.3% of patients with only PNES and in 91.9% of those with both PNES and organic epilepsy [12].

There are two major presentations of functional neurological symptoms:

1. Conversion disorder (CD), also called Briquet's or hysteria, is a disease of young women associated with psychological trauma and the patients are seemingly unaware of the syndrome. Other terms include functional neurological syndromes (preferred term) and somatoform disorders.
2. Malingering syndrome of men which, to the best of our assessments, appears deliberate and insightful, and sometimes presenting with Münchausens syndrome as well as hypochondriasis and sociopathy.

Conversion disorders frequently include symptoms of motor function, sensory function tremor, dystonia, and pseudo-epilepsy mimicking neurological syndromes. Contrary to malingering or factitious disorders, conversion symptoms are unintentional and not deliberately produced. The differential diagnosis is extensive and needs rigorous consideration (Table 3.5).

When faced with the possibility of conversion disorder, specific motor and sensory tests are needed to complement the history in ascertaining a more precise diagnosis. During the clinical examination it may at times be necessary to engage in what is termed "clinical subterfuge" for the evaluation of potential functional sensory impairment (Table 3.6).

An important test of motor examination is to perform Hoover's test (Hoover 1908) [13, 14], applicable to the leg, however. This is probably the best known and touted as one of the more reliable signs to assess conversion type paresis or plegia.

This is a two-step test. For example, with right leg weakness as a presentation, the examiner's hand is placed under the heel of the patient's right foot. The patient is then then requested to apply downward pressure with the right leg, that is performing hip extension. In both organic and functional plegias, no pressure will be appreciated by the examiner's hand. In the second step, with the hand remaining under the right heel, the patient is instructed to lift the left leg off the bed (hip flexion) against resistance of the examiner's other hand. In the case of functional

Table 3.6 Motor and sensory tests in conversion disorder	Motor tests
	1. Hoover's sign
	2. Hoover's arm sign
	3. Sonoo abductor sign
	4. Co-contraction sign
	5. Sternocleidomastoid sign
	Sensory tests
	1. Reporting sensory testing perception with "yes" and "no"
	2. Sensory testing of fingers with hands are in contorted positions
	3. Midline sensory splitting
	4. Slanting and horizontal truncal sensory levels
	5. Glove and stocking, glove-ankle-sock distributions
	6. SHOT syndrome detection

weakness, a downward pressure will be evident from the right leg due to the involuntary hip extension, which is also termed "associated movements" [13–15].

With flexion of the outstretched arm (unaffected arm) against resistance, this would normally result in an involuntary extension of the opposite or "paretic" arm. What may also be noted is that with shoulder adduction in one arm, the opposite arm will also adduct in patients only with functional paresis of upper limb. This does not occur with organic weakness [15].

The patient is instructed to abduct one leg at a time with resistance provided by the examiner by placing the hands on the outside of both legs. With organic weakness, when the weak leg is abducted, the normal leg remains stable. In CD, a hyperadduction occurs. This test is more objective due to the visual component provided [16].

This is easily noted when testing biceps contraction with the triceps also contracting as in the case of CD weakness. The contraction of the antagonist muscles can also be felt when testing the agonist muscle.

Because sternocleidomastoid muscles have bilateral innervation, in those with organic hemiparesis, no sternocleidomastoid weakness is evident. This is not appreciated in those with CD-related weakness [17].

1. Sensory testing may be employed in patients with the command, say "yes" when you feel and "no" if you do not. The patient may respond "no," when they do not "feel" so.
2. Checking sensation when hands are in contorted positions with fingers intertwined is sometimes useful, causing difficulty in determining which finger belongs to which hand. This may be useful in assessment of "functional analgesia."
3. Midline sensory loss splitting assessment. With functional sensory impairment, the deficit is usually in a hemi-anesthetic pattern, which is mostly left sided. With organic sensory loss, the deficit does not precisely extend to the midline.

The sensation usually begins several millimeters before the midline. In those with functional sensory loss, a typically abrupt delineation at the midline occurs which may also involve the vibration modality.

4. Truncal sensory levels may be recorded to slant downward when tested from back to front in organic lesions. In CD, the functional level is usually found to be strictly horizontal.

5. Glove and stocking-level distributions may be informative. When the impairment in the legs reaches the knee level, it should be at approximately the wrist level in the upper limbs.

With CD, the deficit may be distal to wrists and ankles, which is known as glove-ankle-sock distribution [18, 19].

No *s*ight in the eye

No *h*earing in the ear

No *o*lfaction in the nose

No *t*ouch sensation on the body

All of these are reported on the same side of the body, which is not neuroanatomically possible [20].

Neuroimaging Functional Imaging Overview and the Importance of Conceiving Disorders in Terms of Network Syndromes

A number of regions are neurobiologically related to the conversion paresis [21]. Abnormalities in neural networks as opposed to specific areas have been reported by various functional imaging (f-MRI, PET, ICNs) studies. Amygdala activation triggered by adverse experiences may be the initial event with subsequent frontal and limbic networks impacted with respect to both perceptual experiences (sensory loss) and movements (weakness). Functional imaging in conversion disorder (CD) patients has also documented a correlation with focal right frontal lobe activation, implying an inhibitory effect on motor or sensory actions [22]. With motor CD, greater functional connectivity by f-MRI was reported between the right amygdala and right supplementary motor region, despite no direct neuroanatomical networks between the supplementary motor area (SMA) and amygdala [23]. The supplementary motor is involved in self-initiated actions and the source of the "Bereitschaftspotential" (readiness potential), a frontal lobe, electrophysiological negative potential that precedes movement by about 1 second [24].

Other brain regions have also been implicated in CD, such as the right temporo-parietal junction (TPJ) with documentation of hypoactivity in CD patients. Decreased activity in the precuneus (medial parietal lobe area) as well as increased supra-marginal gyrus activity (lateral parietal lobe) have been reported (Fig. 3.1), The lateral parietal lobe in conjunction with the supplementary motor area are the regions mediating planning of motor control. In summary, motor conversion disorder is associated with amygdala activation (stress, threats, adverse experiences) with downstream influences on the supplementary motor area (SMA), the site of motor plans, motor initiation, and non-conscious response inhibition [25–27].

References

1. Marcantonio ER. Delirium in hospitalized older adults. N Engl J Med. 2017;377:1456–66.
2. Edmonds EC, Delano-Wood L, Jak AJ, et al. "Missed" mild cognitive impairment: high false-negative error rate based on conventional diagnostic criteria. J Alzheimer's Dis. 2016;52:685–91. https://doi.org/10.3233/JAD-150986.
3. Petersen RC, Lopez O, Armstrong MJ, et al. Practice guideline update summary: mild cognitive impairment. Neurology. 2018;90:126–35.
4. O'Donnell MJ, et al. Risk factors for ischemic and intracerebral hemorrhagic stroke in 22 countries (Interstroke study): a case control study. Lancet. 2010;376:112–23.
5. Viswanathan A, Rocca WA, Tzourio C. Vascular risk factors and dementia: how to move forward? Neurology. 2009;72:368–74.
6. Fiturria-Medina Y, Sotero RC, Toussaint PJ et al. Early role of vascular dysregulation on late onset Alzheimer's disease based on multifactorial data driven analysis. Nat Commun 2016;7:11934:1–14. https://doi.org/10.1038/ncomms11934; www.nature.com/naturecommunications.
7. Bettcher BM. Normal aging of the frontal lobes. In: Miller BL, Cummings JL, editors. The human frontal lobes. London: The Guilford Press; 2018.
8. Bredesen DA. Reversal of cognitive decline. A novel therapeutic program. Aging. 2014;6:707–16.
9. Bell V, Oakley DA, Halligan PW, Deeley Q. Dissociation in hysteria and hypnosis: evidence from cognitive neuroscience. J Neurol Neurosurg Psychiatry. 2011;82(3):332–9. https://doi.org/10.1136/jnnp.2009.199158. Epub 2010 Sep 30
10. Carson AH, Brown R, David AS et al. Functional (conversion) Neurological Syndromes: research since the millennium Journal of Neurology, Neurosurgery & Psychiatry. 2012;83:842–50.
11. Stone J, Warlow C, Sharpe M. The symptom of functional weakness: a controlled study of 107 patients. Brain. 2010;132:2878–88.
12. Reuber M. The etiology of psychogenic non-epileptic seizures: toward a biopsychosocial model. Neurol Clin. 2009;27:909e24.
13. Hoover CF. A new sign for the detection of malingering and functional paresis of the lower extremities. JAMA. 1908;51:746–7.
14. Koehler PJ, Okun MS. Important observations prior to the description of the Hoover sign. Neurology. 2004;63:1693–7.
15. Mehndiratta MM, Kumar M, Nayak R, Garg H, Pandey S. Hoover's sign: clinical relevance in neurology. J Postgrad Med. 2014;60:297–9.
16. Sonoo M. Abductor sign: a reliable new sign to detect unilateral non-organic paresis of the lower limb. J Neurol Neurosurg Psychiatry. 2004;75:121–5.
17. Diukova GM, Stolajrova AV, Vein AM. Sternocleidomastoid (SCM) muscle test in patients with hysterical and organic paresis. J Neurol Sci. 2001;187(Suppl 1):S108.
18. Stone J, Zeman A, Sharpe M. Functional weakness and sensory disturbance. J Neurol Neurosurg Psychiatry. 2002;73:241–5.
19. Vuilleumier P, Chicherio C, Assal F, Schwartz S, Slosman D, Landis T. Functional neuroanatomical correlates of hysterical sensorimotor loss. Brain. 2001;124:1077–90.
20. Campbell WW, De Jong RN. The neurologic examination. New York: Lippincott Williams and Wilkins; 2005.

21. Van Beilen M, de Jong BM, Gieteling EW, Renken R, Leenders KL. Abnormal parietal function in conversion paresis. PLoS One. 2011;6(10):e25918.
22. Marshall JC, Halligan PW, Fink GR, Wade DT, Frackowiak RS. The functional anatomy of a hysterical paralysis. Cognition. 1997;64(1):B1–8.
23. Groenewegen HJ, Wright CI, Uylings HB. The anatomical relationships of the prefrontal cortex with limbic structures and the basal ganglia. J Psychopharmacol. 1997;11:99–106.
24. Shibasaki H, Hallett M. What is the Bereitschaftspotential? Clin Neurophysiol. 2006;117:2341–56.
25. Voon V, Brezing C, Gallea C, et al. Emotional stimuli and motor conversion disorder. Brain. 2010;133:1526–36.
26. Kanaan RA, Craig TK, Wessely SC, et al. Imaging repressed memories in motor conversion disorder. Psychom Med. 2007;69:202–5.
27. Arnsten AFT. Stress signaling pathways that impair prefrontal cortex structure and function. Nat Rev Neurosci. 2009;10:410–22.

Chapter 4
Cognitive Reserve and Its Implications in Cognitive and Behavioral Testing

Cognitive reserve (CR) may mask brain pathology until late in certain brain disease processes. People with similar cognitive impairment may have markedly different pathology of Alzheimer's disease, for example, depending on their degree of brain and cognitive reserve. Because of the cognitive reserve hypothesis, clinical examination alone cannot discern cognitive impairment. The cognitive reserve hypothesis proposes that people with similar cognitive impairments or even no impairment at all may nevertheless have rampant Alzheimer pathology. Hence, clinical psychometric testing is unlikely to reliably diagnose many people that may benefit from specific disease therapies. Metabolic testing with positron emission tomography (PET) brain scanning is known to improve diagnosis and extend the window of AD diagnosis into the mild clinical and even preclinical phase. Another facet of complexity concerns the increasing number of classic dementia presentations being encountered that are caused by other treatable and at times completely reversible medical and neurological diseases. Most of these can be identified by the proposed cognitive and behavioral evaluations. CR is regarded as interceding between pathology and the degree and timing of clinical presentations of cognitive and behavioral impairment (Fig. 4.1). The discrepancy between brain pathology and cognitive status can be attributed to adequate CR.

Contemporary studies reported during 2019 by Villeneuve et al. and Xu et al. revealed that a CR score can be derived from age, education, and risk factor adjusted measures of education, lifelong cognitive activity, and social activity. A higher reserve combination was associated with a 40% reduction in dementia in highest quartile tested by Xu et al. and delayed the onset of dementia by ~7 years. In addition, there was a dose effect reported in the group within the mid-quartile showing a ~20% reduction in dementia [1, 2].

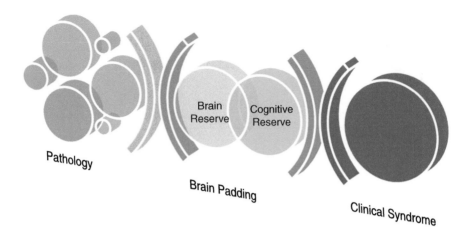

Fig. 4.1 Cognitive reserve: a moderator between underlying pathology and clinical presentation

Epidemiological Studies

In general, studies have shown an approximate 35% of AD risk that is potentially modifiable. For example, a lifetime exposure to advanced education and higher occupational attainment in addition to cognitively stimulating activities is associated with overall reduced risk of Alzheimer's disease. Years of education with increased rates of literacy were associated with a slower decline in memory, executive function, and language skills. Studies from many different parts of the world have shown that a range of different activities lead to the development of cognitive reserve and are as follows:

- Traveling, doing "odd jobs," and knitting were associated with a lower risk of incident dementia in a French study [3].
- Community activities and gardening were protective for incident dementia in a Chinese study [4].
- Having an extensive social network was protective for developing incident dementia in a Swedish study [5].
- A study of an elderly population with high leisure activity yielded a 38% lower risk of dementia in a New York city study [6].
- In a prospective study of 801 non-demented Catholic nuns, brothers, and priests on follow-up, a 1 score increase in intellectual activity was associated with a 33% decrease in AD development [7].
- In a study of ethnically diverse, non-demented NYC elders, with any level of clinical cognitive impairment, underlying AD pathology was more advanced in those with estimated CR [8].

Autopsy Studies

A number of autopsy reports have shown individual differences in how much brain pathology people can tolerate before manifesting with cognitive impairments. About one-third of people who are cognitively normal have neuropathological criteria for AD [9]. Cognitive reserve is not only important for mitigating dementia with the following conditions also potentially benefiting:

- Cognitive vascular disease
- Parkinson's disease
- Frontotemporal lobe disorder
- Progressive Lewy body disease
- Multiple sclerosis
- HIV dementia
- Traumatic brain injury
- Depression, anxiety

The Neurobiology of Cognitive Reserve (Fig. 4.2)

Yakov Stern's very insightful model postulates the following:

- Brain reserve capacity (hardware) concerns brain size, neural count, or synapse count.
- Cognitive reserve (software) – whereby the brain actively attempts to minimize brain damage, using inherent cognitive processing or other compensatory approaches. Hence, people with higher education and occupational attainment are therefore able to withstand brain damage better.
- Neural reserve concerns cerebral networks that may be more robust and less susceptible to disruptive pathology by being composed of more efficient and

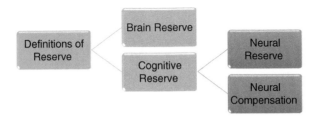

Fig. 4.2 Brain reserve and cognitive reserve. (1) Neural reserve; preexisting differences in neural efficiency or capacity. (2) Neural compensation; individual differences in ability for new compensatory responses to the effects of pathology

resilient networks. Neural compensation is thought to be a feature of some people who may simply be more adaptive in using existing neural compensatory mechanisms [10].

More recent insights include both hippocampal neurogenesis as a more recently evolved trait for cognitive adaptability for specific environmental challenges [11] and the human microbiome with its microbiota influencing brain and behavior [12].

Clinical studies (neurologically healthy older adults (n = 717) from a community-based study) using the vascular model for example have shown that increased white matter hyperintensity (WMH) volume (leukoaraiosis) was associated with poorer cognition and higher cognitive and brain reserves were associated with better cognition. In addition, those with higher reserve tolerated greater amounts of pathology compared to the group with lower reserve. For any given level of cognitive function, those with higher reserve had more WMH pathology, implying they are better at coping with pathology than those with lower reserve [13]. A number of factors can impact CR including microbiome health and cerebrovascular health (Figs. 4.3 and 4.4).

A neural substrate of cognitive reserve has recently been demonstrated by connectomal imaging. The left frontal hub connectivity seems particularly important. Elevated global left frontal cortex (gLFC) connectivity, a reduction of entorhinal tau PET measured levels which impacts episodic memory in older adults was reported.

Fig. 4.3 Cognitive reserve and leukoaraiosis. (Brickman [18])

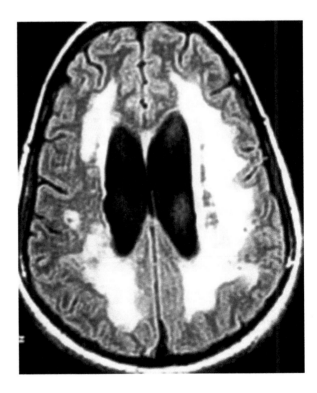

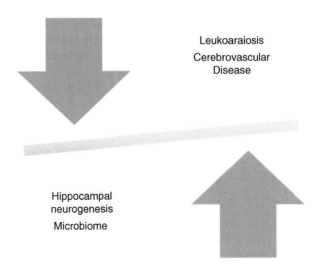

Fig. 4.4 Neurobiology of cognitive reserve candidates

Both gLFC and higher levels of left frontal cortex connectivity were associated with more durability against the adverse effects of entorhinal tau deposition which in turn impacting memory capacity. This was supported by another similar study [14, 15].

Clinical Assessment: Measures of Cognitive Reserve Proxy Variables

- Education
- Socioeconomic status
- Degrees of literacy – regarded as a better marker than education or years of occupation
- Intelligence quotient
- Other cognitive measures (WAIS 33 vocabulary test)
- Cognitive reserve indices [16, 17]

What This Means for Clinical Evaluation of People with Mild Cognitive Impairment and Dementia

Different people with the same clinical cognitive evaluation may have markedly divergent levels of underlying neurodegenerative disease pathology whether due to amyloid, tau, Lewy bodies, or TDP 43. This has profound clinical implications for diagnosing MCI and dementias in the preclinical stages. Clinical evaluation alone remains inadequate as a measure of patient's true status and neuroimaging (PET brain scanning, intrinsic connectivity network testing), and cerebrospinal fluid biomarkers (tau, amyloid) are needed to complement the assessment. Perhaps even more important is the prospect of some degree of reversibility or improvement in a person's cognition by key life exposures such as engaging in cognitive-stimulating leisure activities, education years, and level of occupation to boost cognitive reserve or brain padding – a true disease-modifying approach.

References

1. Villeneuve S. Lifespan cognitive reserve – a secret to coping with neurodegenerative pathology. JAMA Neurol. 2019;76:1145–6.
2. Xu H, Yang R, Qi X, et al. Association of lifespan cognitive reserve indicator with dementia risk in the presence of brain pathologies. JAMA Neurol. 2019;76:1184–91.
3. Fabriguole C, et al. Social and leisure activities and risk of dementia. A prospective longitudinal study. J Am Geriatric Soc. 1995;43:485–90.
4. Wang H-X, et al. Late life engagement in social and leisure activities is associated with a decreased risk of dementia: a longitudinal study from the Kungsholmen project. Am J Epidemiol. 2002;155:1081–7.
5. Fratiglioni L, et al. Influence of social network on occurrence of dementia: a community based longitudinal study. Lancet. 2000;355:1315–9.
6. Scarmeas N, Levy G, Tang MX, Manly J, Stern Y. Influence of leisure activity on the incidence of Alzheimer disease. Neurology. 2001;57:2236–42.
7. Wilson RS, et al. Participation in cognitively stimulating activities and in risk of incident Alzheimer's disease. J Am Med Assoc. 2002;287:742–8.
8. Manly JJ, et al. Cognitive decline and literacy among ethnically diverse elders. J Geriatric Psychiatry Neurol. 2005;18:213–7.
9. Schneider JA, et al. The neuropathology of probable Alzheimer disease and mild cognitive impairment. Ann Neurol. 2009;66:200–8.
10. Stern Y. Cognitive reserve. Alzheimer Dis Assoc Disord. 2006;20:112–7.
11. Kemperman G. New neurons for survival of the fittest. Nat Neurosci Rev. 2012;13:727–36.
12. Cryan JF, Dinan TG. Mind altering micro-organisms: the impact of the gut microbiota on brain and behavior. Nat Neurosci Rev. 2012;13:701–12.
13. Zhuang L, Sachdev PS, Tollor JN, Kochan NA, Reppermund S, Brodaty H, Wen W. Microstructural white matter changes in cognitively normal individuals at risk of amnestic MCI. Neurology. 2012;79:748–54.
14. Neitzel J, Franzmeier N, Rubinski A, et al. Left frontal connectivity attenuates the adverse effect of entorhinal tau pathology on memory. Neurology. 2019;93:e347–57.
15. Franzmeier N, Düzel E, Jessen F, et al. Left frontal hub connectivity delays cognitive impairment in autosomal-dominant and sporadic Alzheimer's disease. Brandweek. 2018;141:1186–200.
16. Nucci M1, Mapelli D, Mondini S. Cognitive Reserve Index questionnaire (CRIq): a new instrument for measuring cognitive reserve. Aging Clin Exp Res. 2012;24(3):218–26.
17. Kartschmit N, Mikolajczy R, Schubert T, Lacruz ME. Measuring Cognitive Reserve (CR) – a systematic review of measurement properties of CR questionnaires for the adult population. PLoS One. 2019;14(8):e0219851.
18. Brickman AM, Siedleck KL, Muraskin J et al. White matter hyperintensities and cognition: testing the reserve hypothesis. Neurobiol Aging 2011;32:1588–98.

Chapter 5
Bedside Mental Status Evaluation: Overview, Coconuts, Cobe-50

Current clinical neuroscientists and their domains of cognitive testing include neurologists, psychiatrists, neuropsychologists, and speech and language clinicians, along with neuro-radiologists providing critical and complementary information of lesion location. All are important to capture the extent and nature of the deficits. For example, any degree of significant aphasia will curtail the number and type of testing that is possible. The abulic spectrum of disorders may severely limit testing and the mild and often covert forms of inattention due minimal hepatic encephalopathy (MHE) with elevated ammonia level precludes in depth neuropsychological assessment. It is not unusual for people with MHE to present because of multiple motor vehicle accidents on account of their inattention. As with most frontal lobe syndromes, the spouse, family, or other informant is most important.

The bedside-type mental status tests have evolved over the past few decades from focusing almost solely on memory testing such as the Delayed Word Recall (DWR) Test [1]. The Blessed Information Memory Concentration Test (BIMC) [2], the Veterans Affairs Medical Center, St Louis University Mental Status examination (VAMC SLUMS) [3] and others such as the Mini-Mental Status Examination (MMSE) [4] were subsequently developed, the latter which included some aspects of language and visuospatial construction evaluation. A degree of executive aspects is captured by the Montreal Cognitive Assessment (MOCA) [5]. More inclusive and broader cognitive domains are features of Kipps and Hodges 12-min cognitive evaluation [6] and the Philadelphia Brief Assessment of Cognition [7]. With the appreciation of the concept of mild behavioral impairment (MBI) becoming prominent, the Addenbrooke's Cognitive Examination-Revised (ACE-R) [8], MBI-C tests [9, 10], the Toronto Cognitive Assessment (TorCA) [11], and the Behavioral Neurological Assessment test were developed [12].

Neuropsychological testing (NPT), for example, generally captures six major domains, providing metric and standardized scores, with some ordinal and numeric. A comprehensive higher cortical functional or mental state evaluation should

© Springer Nature Switzerland AG 2020
M. Hoffmann, *Clinical Mentation Evaluation*,
https://doi.org/10.1007/978-3-030-46324-3_5

Table 5.1 Some of the tests currently in use

1. MMSE
2. MOCA
3. The Philadelphia brief assessment of cognition
4. Addenbrooke's cognitive examination
5. TORCA
6. Kipps and Hodges 12-min cognitive examination
Behavioral tests
7. FRSBE [13]
8. FBI [14]
9. FAB [15]
10. BRIEF [16]
11. EXIT [17]
12. Iowa gambling test [18]
13. Daphne [19]
14. BNA [12]
15. MBI-C [9]

include a process of interrogating not only cognitive but also conative (motivational aspects) and behavioral sequelae to nervous system disruption. Recent research and reviews by Ismail et al. emphasized the need to include mild behavioral impairment (MBI) assessment together with the assessment of mild cognitive impairment (MCI). Not only may they coexist in most people with symptoms but also MBI may precede MCI by many years and may be the sole manifestation as indeed they are with frontotemporal degenerations. MBI may also be the reason that NPT cannot proceed or be severely curtailed. In addition, many syndromes may not be amenable to neuropsychological testing because of the time factors (2–8 h), sometimes a significant aphasia or an inability of patients to cooperate due to inattention and abulia that are themselves part of the neurological deficit.

A bedside screening test should be just that. The total score of brief mental tests is not as important as delineating the individual deficits which then can be focused on with metric tests. As with the NIH stroke scale, a score of 0 is normal and any value of 1 or more abnormal. The bedside mental state tests presented are viewed in a similar light. Even when the so-called normal people score 1 or several points worth of abnormality, they are still abnormal. An overarching review of the principal cognitive and behavioral domains is to detect any particular deficit that can then be used as a springboard to enlist focused metric tests and monitor the particular group of deficits over time. These will be discussed in more detail in the subsequent chapters that discuss the large-scale clinical neural networks and their corresponding intrinsic connectivity webs or connectomes. However, with identification of significant behavioral impairments using one of the bedside screening tests, further delineation with standardized metric tests using those in Table 5.1 can be employed.

A Proposal for a Practical Neurological, Time-Oriented, Hierarchical Assessment

Depending on the patient's presentation, this may be a code situation, an urgent scenario or one that may allow more delayed evaluation:

Hyperacute	0–6 h
Acute	>6 h to 1 week
Subacute	1 week to 3 months
Chronic	>3 months

Hyperacute and Acute Presentations

These are generally amenable to brief evaluations. Altered mental status, delirium, or subarachnoid hemorrhage is usually evaluated according to AAOx3 (awake, alert, orientated to person place and time). If patient cooperation is sufficient, a 5- or 10-min battery of testing is often possible. Depending on the diagnoses, disease-specific scales are often required for subsequent management and monitoring including the NIH stroke scale, the Hunt and Hess scale in patients with subarachnoid hemorrhage, or the Glasgow coma scale in patients with various degrees of confusion and obtundation. With more time available, improvement in clinical status, and degree of patient cooperation, the time constraints of testing generally allow for more detailed, informative, and also metric testing.

Hyperacute and Acute Presentations

- 1 min AAOx3 or 5 min
- The author's recommendation: High hub value screen Cobe 20 (*co*gnitive and *b*ehavioral *e*valuation) (see below).

Subacute Presentations

- MOCA, MMSE
- The author's recommendation is the 10–15 min Cobe 50 (*co*gnitive and *b*ehavioral *e*valuation) (see below)

Chronic Presentations

- Any of the tests mentioned in Table 5.1 according to diagnoses, time constraints
- The authors recommendation is the 15–20 min Coconuts (see below) and/ or CNS-VS
- If indicated, 2–8 h NPT

The Author's Approach to Cognitive and Behavioral Testing: Using Coconuts, Cobe 20, Cobe 50

The Coconuts test [20] was developed because of the recognition that cognitive syndromes (CS) and behavioral syndromes after stroke were important to measure and monitor for the management and assessment of emerging therapies. By incorporating known behavioral neurological as well as neuropsychiatric syndromes with commonly administered bedside cognitive assessments, a validated "comprehensive cognitive neurological test in stroke" (Coconuts) was developed and administered in patients within the first month of stroke presentations. Validity testing was performed including sensitivity, specificity, negative and positive predictive values and compared to brain neuroimaging with MRI scans for diagnosis of stroke. Discriminant validity, construct validity, and inter-rater reliability were evaluated. The overall sensitivity of the Coconuts scale was 91% and specificity 35%, positive predictive value 88%, and negative predictive 41% versus stroke lesions detected using MRI (DWI or FLAIR). Discriminant validity by comparison to normal subjects and the stroke group study was tested and a normal Coconuts score of 1.9 (SD 1.6) was attained; hence, a score of >3.5 was determined to be abnormal. Coconuts subtest scores were also determined. For these subscales, abnormal scores were defined as mean +1 SD. The mean memory score was 0.6 (SD 0.67), frontal network score 0.8 (SD 1.1), attention and concentration score 0.13 (SD 0.43), visuospatial score 0.3 (SD 0.5), and complex visual processing score 0.1 (SD 0.3). The other subscale scores, for orientation, language, praxis, emotion, neglect, anosognosia, prosody and delusional misidentification syndromes were determined and the mean score for these was 0. Hence, any error was recorded as abnormal. Construct validity was determined for the domains of frontal networks, language, right hemisphere, hippocampal limbic, and complex visual processing networks compared to the corresponding standardized neuropsychological tests. Interrater reliability was excellent (kappa value 0.94). The mean examination timing in normal volunteers was recorded at 13.4 min (SD 2.4).

Although the stroke pathophysiological model was used, the study embraced an extensive collection of cognitive and behavioral syndromes that are also present in many other syndromes and conditions. As the brain lesion localization is no longer challenging today due to the widespread use of multi-modality MR or CT imaging, the more relevant challenge remains in ascertaining the nature and degree of neurological deficit that allow insights into etiopathogenesis as well as more precise deficit monitoring in response to treatments. Hence, Coconuts was considered both a valid and practical test allowing a comprehensive evaluation of currently known cognitive, behavioral neurological, and neuropsychiatric syndromes.

Derivatives of the Coconuts were developed for the purposes of adapting to clinical situations where much briefer scales are suitable. The Cobe 20 (Appendix 2) and Cobe 50 (Appendix 3) versions of the Coconuts have the scoring system reversed to a maximum score of 20 or 50, respectively. The purpose of these two screening tests is not to arrive at a normal score but to detect areas of deficit, with the numeric value of the impaired domain then being used for tracking improvement or deterioration. The Cobe 20 high value hub approach was supplemented because of our recent understanding of connectomal network susceptibility of the high value hubs (attention, executive function, working memory, episodic memory) that are invariably involved in most, if not all, neurological disorders [21].

Appendix 1: COCONUT: Comprehensive Cognitive Neurological Test

Name	Gender		Age
Education years (schooling, college, other)	----		
Handedness (Epworth scale) circle	Right/left/ambidextrous		
Cognitive risk factors (circle). Family history of Alzheimer's, head trauma			
Vascular risk factors. Hypertension, diabetes mellitus, dyslipidemia, smoking, ethanol abuse homocysteine elevation, cardiac disease, atrial fibrillation, coronary artery disease, valvular heart disease, patent foramen ovale, dilated cardiac chamber, leukoaraiosis, BMI ≥ 30			
Neuropsychiatric history (DSM V) circle. Depression, anxiety, obsessive compulsive disorder, substance abuse			

General Attentional Systems

1. *Orientation* 5 items – Score 1 for each error, 0 is normal	
Date (3 for day, month, year), day of week (1), place hospital (or clinic) (1)	/5
2. *Attention and calculation* – Score 1 for each error, 0 is normal	
5 serial 7's, if unable double to 128	/5

Left Hemisphere Network for Language, Gerstmann's, and Angular Gyrus Syndromes

3. *Speech and language* – Score 1 for each error, 0 is normal	
Naming: Name 3 objects (pen, watch, ID card) and name 3 colors	/6
Fluency: Grade as fluent (0), non-fluent (1), mute (2)	/2
Comprehension: Close your eyes, squeeze my hand. Score 1 for each failure	/2
Repetition: "Today is a sunny and windy day." No word repeated (2), partial (1), all (0)	/2
Write a sentence. What is your job? Must contain subject and verb and makes sense	/3
Reading: "Close your eyes." No words read (2), partial (1), or all words (0)	/2
4. *Motor speech*	
Dysarthria. During interview, are words slurred? Nil (0), mild slurring 1, marked slurring (2)	/2
Hypophonia. Normal (0), voice softer than normal (1), very low volume, barely audible (2)	/2
5. *Praxis*	
Rating scale: Impaired 1, unable 2, smooth execution 0	
Melokinetic. Thumb – finger opposition test compare R + L (only if ≥4/5 power)	/2
Buccolingual. Licks your lips, blows up your cheeks	/2
Ideomotor apraxia. Clumsy action with pen or eating utensils	/2
Ideational. Folds piece of paper in half, writes your name, and places inside a file or book	/2
6. *Right, left, and body part orientation*	
Left pointing finger on right ear (one point for each error)	/2

Hippocampal Limbic Network for Memory and Emotion

7. *Memory* – Score 1 for each error, 0 is normal	
Short-term memory: Registers five words (orange, ocean, courage, rapid, building)	
Test recall at 5 min. Score 1 for each omission	/5
Remote memory: Recites last 3 presidents or 3 important personal dates (graduations)	/3
8. Emotions	
Lability – Laughs or cries easily, out of context. Rarely (1), sometimes (2)	
Frequently (3), never (0)	/3
Geschwind-Gastaut syndrome: Stroke or new lesion induced with new evidence of viscous personality, metaphysical pre-occupation, and altered physiological drives	
(i) Viscous personality: One or more of the following. Circumstantiality in speech, over-inclusive verbal discourse, excessive detail of information, stickiness of thought processes, interpersonal adhesiveness, prolongation of interpersonal encounters, and hypergraphia	
(ii) Metaphysical pre-occupation: One or more of the following: Overly philosophical pre-occupation, nascent and excessive intellectual interests in religion, philosophy and moral issues.	
(iii) Altered physiological drives: One or more of the following: Hyposexuality, aggression, and fear	
Scoring: Two out of three components required for diagnosis	
Score as 3 components (3), 2 components (2), 1 component (1), nil (0)	/3

Prefrontal Network and Subcortical Network for Executive Function and Comportment

9. *Serial motor programming: Luria motor sequence test* (fist-palm-hand). Demonstrate sequence until patient able to replicate. Then do 5 cycles	
Score 1 for each error in sequence	/5
10. *Word fluency.* Says as many words starting with S in 1 min (no names or places)	
Grading: >15 (0), 13–15 (1), 10–12 (2), 7–9 (3), 4–6 (4), 0–3 (5)	/5
11. *Environmental autonomy* (imitation and utilization behavior)	
Imitation behavior. Maintaining eye contact, pats side of examiner's face, and then claps the hands without suggesting patient to follow suit	
Scoring: Copies all actions spontaneously (2,) copies some (1), nil (0)	/2
Utilization behavior: Places three objects in front of patient, key, cell phone, and pen	
Scoring: Unsolicited manipulation of 1 or 2 objects (1) or all (2)	/2
12. *Interference and inhibitory control* (Go-No-Go paradigm)	
If examiner taps once, raise your finger; if examiner taps twice, do not raise finger	
Do three cycles: 1-1-2, 1-2-1, 2-2-1. Score 1 for each incorrect response	/3
13. *Abulia.* Poverty of action and speech. Grade as marked 2, somewhat 1, nil 0	/2
14. *Disinhibition:* Comments or actions during interview. Occasional 1, frequent 2, nil 0	/2
15. *Impersistence.* Discontinues Luria's sequences, despite repeated coaxing x 3	/1
16. *Perseveration.* During Luria sequence test, duplicates same hand position	/1

Dorsal Right Parieto-Frontal Network for Visuospatial Function, Attention, Emotion, and Prosody

17. *Visuospatial*	
Copy a 2D image of examiner's drawn flower. Impaired 1, marked 2, nil 0	/2
Copy a 3D image representation of examiner's cube. Impaired 1, marked 2, nil 0	/2
18. *Neglect syndromes*	
Tactile. Simultaneous stimulation of both arms. Omission of one side score 1	/1
Auditory. Simultaneous stimulation of both ears. Omission of one side score 1	/1
Visual. Simultaneous stimulation of both fields. Omission of one side score 1	/1

Motor neglect. Bisect 10 cm line. More than 1/4 (2.5 cm) distance from midline, score 1	/1
19. *Anosognosia*	
Recognizes weakness 0, underestimation 1, or complete denial of deficit or illness 2	/2
20. *Prosody*	
As per family, speech has become flat or monotone, then score 1; if not score 0	/1
Cannot comprehend different intonations (happy/sad), then score 1; if not score 0	/1
Cannot repeat altered intonation (happy/sad), then score 1; if not score 0	/1

Ventral Occipitotemporal Network for Object and Face Recognition

21. Complex visual processing (a score of 0 is normal)	
Object agnosia. Cannot name 3 objects by visual inspection, but can by touch or sound	/3
Achromatopsia. Cannot distinguish 2 different hues or colors. Score 1 for each error	/2
Simultanagnosia. CTPT – identifies all 3 persons (score 0, 1, 2, 3) or analog time telling (m/h/sec)	/3
Optic ataxia. Touches examiners finger under visual guidance. Score 1 for a miss	/1
Optic apraxia. Looks left, right, up, or down to command. Score 1 for any error	/1
Prosopagnosia: Does not recognize family or friends by visual appearance, score 1	/1
Line orientation. Draws 45° and 30° lines. Match 2 lines to figure. Score 1 for error	/2
Subjective report of impaired motion perception (akinetopsia). Score 1 if present	/1
Subjective report of depth perception impairment (astereopsis). Score 1 if present	/1
Hallucinations. Simple (colors, shapes), complex (scenes, people, animals), or experiential (out of body experience or autoscopy). Score 1 if present	/1
Illusions of shape or size. Score 1 if present. Example macropsia or micropsia	/1
Denial of cortical blindness (Anton's syndrome). Score 1 if present	/1

Syndromes with Ill-Defined Neural Networks

22. *Disconnection syndromes* Score 1 if present, 0 if absent	
Alien hand syndrome. The one hand interferes with the other during routine tasks	/1
Alexia without agraphia. Can write but cannot read	/1
Pure word deafness. Hears environmental sounds but not spoken speech	/1
23. *Delusional misidentification syndromes (incorrect ID of people or place). If present 1*	
Reduplicative paramnesia (the person thinks that they are geographically in a different location such as at the office or at home, when in fact they may be lying in a hospital bed)	/1
Capgras or Fregoli syndrome. Familiar people appear strange or vice versa	/1

Miscellaneous Syndromes

Amusia – May be receptive (poor appreciation of music) or expressive (where no longer able to play or sing). Score 1 if either is present	/1
Allesthesia. During neurological examination, transfers perceived tactile stimuli from left to the right or vice versa	/1
Autoscopy. During interview, reports out of body experience	/1
Synesthesia. Activation of one sensory system induces perceived sensation in another	/1
Geographical disorientation or Topographical Disorientation	/1
Cognitive score total	---

CTPT cookie theft picture test

Appendix 2: Cobe 20: High Value Hub Screen

1. Language: Ability to communicate and engage in cognitive testing	
Comprehension: Closes your eyes and makes a fist; if both correct score 1	1/1
Fluency: If no hesitations or paraphasias, naming cell phone, pen; if correct score 1	1/1
2. Attention, abulia	
Abulia: Poverty of speech, actions, slowed instruction processing. If no abulia score 1	1/1
Attention: Orientation 5 items (date, day of week, place)	5/5
3. Executive function	
Serial 7's, 1007 test (93,86,79,72,65)	5/5
Phonemic fluency words beginning with "F" in 1 min; if ≥12 score 1	1/1
4. Working memory	
Working memory: Digits 5 back, example: 85410...01458; if correct score 1	1/1
5. Episodic verbal memory	
Learn/register words: Ocean, orange, courage, building, rapid, recall at 5 min	5/5
Total score	/20

Appendix 3: Cobe 50: A Brief Mental Status Test, a Precision Tool for an Individual (n = 1). Score 1 for Each Correct Item

Cognitive domains	
Attention	
1. Orientation 5 items (date, day of week, place)	5/5
2. Serial 7's, 1007 test (93,86,79,72,65)	5/5
Language, praxis, acquired cultural circuits	
1. Fluency: If no hesitations, paraphasias, stuttering during discourse, score 1	1/1
2. Comprehension: Closes your eyes and makes a fist; if both correct score 1	1/1
3. Repetition "Today is a sunny and windy day"	1/1
4. Naming: 5 items: Cell phone, pen, ID card, computer keyboard, magazine	5/5

Cognitive domains	
5. No dysarthria or hypophonia	1/1
6. Reading/writing: Reads and executes: What is your job? (has subject, verb, makes sense)	1/1
7. Praxis: Shows hand position when using a pair of scissors	1/1
Executive function	
1. Phonemic fluency words beginning with "F" in 1 min; if ≥12 score 1	1/1
2. Semantic fluency, animal naming; if ≥16 score 1	1/1
3. Working memory: Digits 5 back, example: 85410…01458; if correct score 1	1/1
4. Luria motor series (fist, palm, hand sequence) do 5 cycles; if all correct score 1	1/1
5. Speed of information processing (short trails test): 1A-2B-3C-4D-5E; if all correct score 1	1/1
Visuospatial	
1. Draws a clock with numbers at 10 past 11; if good copy, score 1	1/1
2. Draws a 3-dimensional (Necker) cube; if good copy, score 1	1/1
Memory	
1. Verbal: Learns to register words: Ocean, orange, courage, building, rapid, recall at 5 min	5/5
2. Nonverbal: Learns to register by copying 5-point star, triangle, cross, recall at 5 min	3/3
3. Remote memory (any 2 personal notable events: school/college graduation, wedding)	2/2
Behavioral domains	
Conation	
1. Abulia: Poverty of speech, actions, slowed processing of instructions. No abulia scores 1	1/1
Disinhibition	
1. Go-No-Go paradigm: Lifts index finger for 1 tap, does not lift for 2 taps; if 5 cycles correct	1/1
2. Disinhibition: Inappropriate joviality, remarks, actions toward others; if absent score 1	1/1
3. Prehension behavior – Maintains attention, pats side of examiner's face, then claps hands without suggesting patient to follow suit; score 0 for no imitation, score 1 if enacts either imitation	1/1
Emotional regulation	
1. Empathy disorders (intrapersonal emotional intelligence)	
Emotional blunting, poor or inappropriate emotion detection; if absent score 1	1/1
4. Sociopathy (interpersonal emotional intelligence)	
Prefers to avoid people, crowds, has become asocial or dysocial; if absent score 1	1/1
5. Emotional lability (involuntary emotional expression disorder (IEED))	
Laughs or cries easily or out of context; if absent score 1	1/1
Independency (ADL)	
Basic: Toilet, feeding, bathing, dressing, continence, transfer; if all intact score 1	1/1
Instrumental: Finances, shopping, medications, driving, meal prep; if all intact score 1	1/1
Cognitive reserve	
Educational level in years, school, college, if 12 or more score 1	1/1
Languages spoken, if 2 or more score 1	1/1
Total	/50

References

1. Knopman DS, Ryberg S. A verbal memory test with high predictive accuracy for dementia of the Alzheimer type. Arch Neurol. 1989;46:141–5.
2. Tariq NT, Chibnall JT, Perry HM III, Morley JE. The Saint Louis university mental status (SLUMS) examination for detecting mild cognitive impairment and dementia is more sensitive than the mini-mental status examination (MMSE) a pilot study. Am J Geriatr Psychiatry. 2006;14(11):900–10.
3. Blessed G, Tomlinson BE, Roth M. The association between quantitative measures of dementia and of senile changes in the cerebral gray matter of elderly subjects. Br J Psychiatry. 1968;114:7970811.
4. Folstein MF, Folstein SE, McHugh PR. "Mini-mental state". A practical method for grading cognitive state of patients for the clinician. J Pyschiatry Res. 1975;12:189–98.
5. Nasreddine ZS, Phillips MA, Bedirian V, Charbonneau S, Whitehead V, Collin I, Cummings JL, Chertkow H. The Montreal cognitive assessment MoCA: a brief screening tool for mild cognitive impairment. J Am Geriatr Soc. 2005;53:695–9.
6. Kipps CM, Hodges JR. Cognitive assessment for clinicians. J Neurol Neurosurg Psychiatry. 2005;76(Suppl I):i22–30. https://doi.org/10.1136/jnnp.2004.059758. Kipps and Hodges 12-minute cognitive examination
7. Libon DJ, Rascovsky K, Gross RG, et al. The Philadelphia Brief Assessment of Cognition (PBAC): a valisdated screening measure for dementia. The Clinical Neuropsychologist 2011; 25(8):1314–30.
8. Mioshi E, Dawson K, Mitchell J, et al. The Addenbrooke's cognitive examination revised (ACE-R): a brief cognitive test battery for dementia screening. Int J Geriatr Psychiatry. 2006;21:1078–85.
9. Ismail Z, Agüera-Ortiz L, Brodaty H, et al. The mild behavioral impairment checklist (MBI-C): a rating scale for neuropsychiatric symptoms in pre-dementia populations. J Alzheimers Dis. 2017;56:929–38.
10. Ismail Z, Smith EE, Geda Y, et al. Neuropsychiatric symptoms as early manifestations of emergent dementia: provisional diagnostic criteria for mild behavioral impairment. Alzheimers Dement. 2016;12(2):195–202.
11. Freedman M, Leach L, Tartaglia MC et al. The Toronto Cognitive Assessment (TorCA): normative data and validation to detect amnestic mild cognitive impairment. Alzheimer's Research and Therapy 2018. https://doi.org/10.1186/s13195-018-0382
12. Darvesh S, Leach L, Black SE, et al. The behavioral neurology assessment. Can J Neurol Sci. 2005;32:167–1.
13. Grace J, Malloy PF. Frontal systems behavior scale. Lutz Florida 2002. PAR.
14. Kertesz A, Davidson W, Fox H. Frontal behavioral inventory: diagnostic criteria for frontal lobe dementia. Can J Neurol Sci. 1997;24:29–36.
15. Dubois B, Slachevsky A, Litvan I, Pillon B. The FAB. A frontal assessment battery at the beside. Neurology. 2000;55:1621–6.
16. Roth RM, Isquith PK, Gioia GA. BRIEF-A. Behavior rating inventory of executive function-adult version. PAR neuropsychological assessment resources Inc. 2005. Lutz Florida.
17. Royall DR, Mahurin RK, Gray KF. Bedside assessment of executive cognitive impairment: the executive interview. J Am Geriatr Soc. 1992;40:1221–6.
18. Bechara A. Iowa gambling test. Psychological Assessment Resources Inc, Lutz Fl 2007.
19. Boutoleau-Bretonnière C, Evrard C, Benoît Hardouin J, et al. DAPHNE: a new tool for the assessment of the behavioral variant of frontotemporal dementia. Dement Geriatr Cogn Disord Extra. 2015;5:503–16.
20. Hoffmann M, Schmitt F, Bromley E. Comprehensive cognitive neurological assessment in stroke. Acta Neurol Scand. 2009;119:162–71.
21. Crossley N, Mechelli A, Scott J, et al. The hubs of the human connectome are generally implicated in the anatomy of brain disorders. Brain. 2014;137:2382–95.

.

Chapter 6
Neuropsychological and Computerized Testing

Neuropsychological testing (NPT) needs to be reserved for patients requiring particularly detailed testing when the symptoms are covert and subtle or where deficits need more precise cognitive appraisal. This applies especially to those with subjective complaints (so- called "worried well"), where close monitoring of cognitive deficits over time is required as with rehabilitation interventions or studies and medicolegal-related assessments. NPT is constrained principally by testing duration and availability. It should also be noted that acute and subacute neurological patients in a tertiary medical setting are often not amenable to NPT as they have obvious significant impairments such as delirium, encephalopathy, global aphasia, severe neglect syndromes or anosognosias, and many common stroke syndromes. In dementia, basic screening is possible, but with mild cognitive impairment, NPT is often indicated. Multiple sclerosis is a good example where elementary neurological deficits such as ophthalmoparesis, ataxia, and sensorimotor impairments may overshadow the majority of patients who have altered cognitive as well as behavioral deficits. Neurotoxicological exposure manifests principally with executive dysfunction where NPT is often useful. Malingering is another good examples of where NPT may play a pivotal role in diagnosis.

The comprehensive AAN report was published with the hopes of guiding the many different clinicians that may be involved with assessing brain function. Some of the most pertinent recommendations including my own are summarized below [1]. Additional historical, neurological, neuroimaging, and laboratory examinations are required for lesion localization, differential diagnosis, pathophysiology, and treatment approaches. Time-honored NPT such as the WAIS-IV and WAIS memory tests remain relatively insensitive to frontal lobe dysfunction, anterior temporal lobe impairments, and various subcortical impairments. A wide range of behavioral impairments that manifest primarily with the numerous facets of disinhibition and abulia may be associated with normal or near normal NPT. On the other hand in those with significant abulia, NPT may be precluded in view of suboptimal cooperation.

© Springer Nature Switzerland AG 2020

M. Hoffmann, *Clinical Mentation Evaluation*,
https://doi.org/10.1007/978-3-030-46324-3_6

Neuropsychological Testing: Validity Measures

- Construct – consistent with theories of cognitive function, do memory tests assess memory?
- Concurrent – do new tests come to same conclusions as older tests?
- Localization – do test results localize focal lesions?
- Diagnostic – do tests accurately diagnose disease?
- Ecologic – do tests results predict real-life performance?
- Criterion validity – associated with known brain damage
- Discriminant validity – test scores differ between various diagnostic groups
- Predictive validity – predictor surgical outcome, for example, epilepsy surgery

Test Reliability

- Interrator
- Intrarator
- Test-retest reliability

Particularly Useful

- When considered for EP surgery
- Litigations question or concerns
- When deficits require quantification
- When deficits are in doubt

Not Particularly Useful for

- Lesion localization
- Etiology
- Differential diagnosis
- Treatment

Disadvantages of NPT

- Time intensive with a typical assessment period of 28 h
- Special equipment/training needed

- Professional/training component demand is high
- Equipment must be secured/testing areas needed
- Moderate expense: typical Neuropsychological evaluation cost ranges from $2000–3000
- Limited accessibility
- Limited access to quality neuropsychological services
- Patient time intensive and demanding. Practice effects are present
- Limited availability of alternate forms
- Limited ecological validity

Common Clinical Misconceptions About NPT

- Although NPT provides the most precise scoring of a large range of standardized testing, it is not intended to provide a diagnosis and not used for localization.
- Detailed testing may lead to overdiagnosis or over-identification of cognitive impairments, and this may lead to an exaggeration of brain dysfunction.

A Selection of Tests Used for Principal NPT Domains

Premorbid Intelligence and Educational Achievement

- NART (National Adult Reading Test)

General Intelligence

- WAIS-IV (Wechsler Adult Intelligence Test) full scale IQ

Attention (Includes Working Memory)

- Digit span forward and back
- Trails A Test or Comprehensive Trail Making Tests 1 and 2
- Letter cancellation tests also cancellation of symbols, colors, or numbers

Language

- Western Aphasia Test-Revised
- Boston Diagnostic Aphasia Examination
- Boston Naming Test

Executive Function

- Verbal fluency
- Animal naming test
- Trails B Test or Comprehensive Trail Making Test 5
- Wisconsin Card Sorting Test
- Stroop test

Memory

- Three Words Three Shapes Test
- Hopkins Verbal Learning Test
- California Verbal Learning Test
- Wechsler Memory Scale
- Rey Auditory Verbal Learning Test

Visuospatial Function

- Rey-Osterrieth Complex Figure Test
- WAIS-IV Block Design Subtest

Computerized Testing (CT)

CT has largely been spearheaded by the specific needs and constraints of institutions such as the NIH, pharmaceutical companies, Department of Defense, aviation, dementia groups, and sports medicine concussion research. Similar to NPT, CT allows for the evaluation of tests according to age, gender, education specific, normative data assessments according to the usual 6 or 7 major cognitive constructs or domains:

1. General cognitive ability (IQ), achievement/academic development
2. Processing speed/psychomotor speed

3. Attention
4. Memory (verbal and visual)
5. Language
6. Visuospatial
7. Executive functions

CT is both complementary and reflects an extension of traditional NPTs. They can be used as both stand-alone tests and also as screening tools for asymptomatic populations, Mild cognitive impairment (MCI) and dementia patients for example which can then trigger" more in depth NPT's evaluation if needed.

Specific Advantages of Computerized Cognitive Assessment

1. There is an increasing need for fast and efficient cognitive testing. For example, in the primary care setting 58% of physicians even find the commonly used MMSE too time consuming to administer [2]
2. NPT is profoundly time intensive and neuropsychological resources are limited.
3. Specific tests used to meaure speed of information processing, working memory, attention and Wisconsin Card Sorting Test are far more efficiently and accurately administered by CT.
4. Relative ease of administration and scoring (1 min to 2 h).
5. Scoring is automated – a significant time saving.
6. Readily available on internet.
7. Relatively inexpensive (30–35 USD per administeration for the CNS-VS test).
8. CT allows real-world setting measurements aided by personal electronic devices and adaptable to almost any environment.
9. Adaptable and flexible for rapid development.
10. Relative short test batteries.
11. Alternate test forms are easily acquired.
12. Can be specifically adapted to a person's specific disease, e.g., multiple sclerosis (MS), traumatic brain injury (TBI), HIV.
13. Large numbers of individuals can be screened.

CT Disadvantages

1. Validity and reliability have been assessed as moderate to good, slightly less than NPT.
2. Potential for high false positives, abuse, and use without adequate training.
3. Personal data vulnerability and data corruption.

A Purview of Some of the Currently Available Computerized Tests

1. King Devick Test – a 1–2 min test, useful in concussion and with suboptimal attention
2. CNS Vital Signs (used in 52 different countries by >10,000 clinicians)
3. NeuroTrax – Mindstreams (particularly useful for portraying 3D evaluations)
4. Automated Neuropsychological Assessment Metrics (ANAM)
5. Cognivue (assesses key cognitive domains, 10-min test, special user interface)
6. CANS-MCI (computer-administered neuropsychological screen)
7. Cambridge Neuropsychological Test Automated Battery (CANTAB)
8. CogSport
9. Headminder
10. ImPACT (concussion test)
11. MicroCog
12. Neurobehavioral Evaluation System 3 (NES 3)

The author has had the most experience with the CNS-VS test (https://www. cnsvs.com). Now in its fourth generation, the program is particularly flexible to the clinical questions asked; for example, different cognitive test domain combinations are used as to whether the diagnosis may be MCI, TBI, MS, ADHD, addiction disorder, and many others. An extensive number of computerized supplementary evaluation scales can be tagged on, such as for depression, anxiety, and Post traumatic stress disorder (PTSD). CNS Vital Signs normative data was gleaned from a sample of 1600 people from ages 8 to 89. The CNS-VS test, is largely self-administered by a dedicated laptop computer. However, occasional supervision and monitoring may be required to make sure that instructions are understood. The cost is 30–35 USD depending on the number of tests purchased and patient security is provided by 128-bit encryption. CNS-VS is available in 60 different languages, and remote testing is easily arranged emphasizing its applicability to telehealth endeavors.

A sample of the easy-to-interpret results page is presented in Fig. 6.1.

Overdiagnosis and Misdiagnosis by NPT and CT

Neuropsychological testing may overestimate the extent of deficit [3, 4]. The profound dissonance that may exist in frontal behavioral impairment and normal or relatively normal cognition frequently escapes detection unless specifically tested for. A Yale University evaluation of clinicians 70 years or older undergoing cognitive screening batteries for the purposes of recredentialing was performed between 2016–2019. Cognitive deficits considered significant in that impairment of their ability to practice was at stake were detected in 8/141 clinicians (12.7%) [5]. More extensive neuropsychological testing was required in 14, and 8/14 clinicians who screened positive were recredentialed implying that the false-positive screening rate was ~57%. The conclusion was that while neuropsychological testing has an

Patient Profile:	Percentile Range				> 74	25 - 74	9 - 24	2 - 8	< 2
	Standard Score Range				> 109	90 - 109	80 - 89	70 - 79	< 70
Domain Scores	Subject Score	Standard Score	Percentile	VI**	Above	Average	Low Average	Low	Very Low
Neurocognition Index (NCI)	NA	94	34	Yes		x			
Composite Memory	105	116	86	Yes	x				
Verbal Memory	54	106	66	Yes		x			
Visual Memory	51	119	90	Yes	x				
Psychomotor Speed	124	67	1	Yes					x
Reaction Time*	643	104	61	Yes		x			
Complex Attention*	12	83	13	Yes			x		
Cognitive Flexibility	44	100	50	Yes		x			
Processing Speed	37	78	7	Yes				x	
Executive Function	46	102	55	Yes		x			
Simple Attention	37	61	1	Yes					x
Motor Speed	86	71	3	Yes				x	

Fig. 6.1 CNS-VS core test domains sample report

important role in such assessments, multiple other sources of information are also to be considered. These may include board certification information, reliability of performance assessments, clinical documentation, simulation testing, and peer assessments. Finally, such programs may also fail to encompass the important recognition of the overall experience as well as accrued wisdom of older physicians [6]. Complementary and paraclinical testing such as evoked potentials, EEG, and neuroradiological examination with MRI or PET scanning may uncover the so-called "silent lesions" that have escaped clinical detection altogether.

References

1. Ferguson JH, Altrocchi P, Brin M, et al. Assessment: neuropsychological testing of adults: considerations for neurologists. Report of the therapeutics and technology assessment Subcommittee of the American Academy of neurology. Neurology. 1996;47:592–9.
2. Tangalos EG, Smith GE, Ivnik RJ, et al. The mini-mental state examination in general medical practice: clinical utility and acceptance. Mayo Clin Proc. 1996;71:829–37.
3. Ana-Claire L, Meyer ACL, Boscardin WJ, Kwasa JK, et al. Is it time to rethink how neuropsychological tests are used to diagnose mild forms of HIV-associated neurocognitive disorders? Impact of false-positive rates on prevalence and power. Neuroepidemiology. 2013;41:208–16. https://doi.org/10.1159/000354629.
4. Lewis MS, Maruff P, Silbert BS, et al. Detection of postoperative cognitive decline after coronary artery bypass graft surgery is affected by the number of neuropsychological tests in the assessment battery. Ann Thoracic Sug. 2006;81(6):2097–104.
5. Cooney L, Balcezak T. Cognitive testing of older clinicians prior to recredentialing. JAMA. 2020;323:179–80.
6. Armstrong KA, Reynolds EE. Opportunities and challenges in valuing and evaluating aging physicians. JAMA. 2020;323:125–6.

Chapter 7
Prefrontal Network for Executive Control of Cognition and Comportment Including the Executive Control, Salience (Ventral Attention) and Semantic Appraisal (SAN) Networks

The cognitive screening tests or neuroimaging will implicate specific brain regions and their circuitry. Various neurological or neuropsychiatric states or syndromes may present in ways that best fit with a network disturbance (for example, Alzheimer's along the default mode network and frontotemporal lobe dementia implicating the salience network). Yet others present with much more focal impairment as with expressive Broca's-type aphasia implicating Brodmann area 44 or Gerstmann's syndrome due to focal stroke or hemorrhage in the inferior parietal lobule or a Wallenberg's syndrome due to lateral medullary infarction. Parkinson's is an example of a state-dependent neurotransmitter-type perturbation secondary to relative dopaminergic deficiency usually ascribed to a substantia nigra degeneration.

The regional frontal anatomical areas are best delineated by the Brodmann areas with corresponding neurophysiological and clinical counterparts (Table 7.1). The principal frontal networks are useful for further localization and understanding. Frontal networks can be described at the macroscopic and mesoscale levels (frontoparietal, frontal subcortical (Table 7.2), fronto-ponto-cerebellar, for example) as well as at microscopic level, such as the state-dependent, ascending neurotransmitter systems from the brainstem and ramifying widely throughout the brain

Table 7.1 Physiology of the prefrontal cortex (PFC) systems, intrinsic functions, and syndromes

Anatomy (BA)	Neurophysiology	Clinical features
1. Medial PFC (24,25,32)	Conation, initiation, energization	Abulia syndromes
2. Orbitofrontal PFC (11,12)	Behavioral/emotional regulation	Disinhibition syndromes
3. Dorsolateral LPFC (46,9)	Task setting (L) and monitoring (R)	Executive dysfunction
4. Frontopolar PFC (10)	Metacognition	Self-awareness, EI, TOM
5. Ventrolateral PFC (44,45,47)	Language processing, inhibition	Expressive aphasia
6. Motor (4)	Skeletomotor	
7. Premotor (6)	Movement planning PMC, SMA	
8. Motor association (8)	Frontal eye fields, SEF	

© Springer Nature Switzerland AG 2020
M. Hoffmann, *Clinical Mentation Evaluation*,
https://doi.org/10.1007/978-3-030-46324-3_7

Table 7.2 Frontal subcortical circuits (channel dependent)

6. Dorsolateral
7. Orbitofrontal
8. Anterior cingulate
9. Oculomotor
10. Motor

Table 7.3 Ascending neurotransmitter, or state-dependent networks and origins

7. Cholinergic projections	From the nucleus basalis of Meynert
8. Histaminergic projections	From the hypothalamus
9. Dopaminergic projections	From the ventral tegmental area
10. Serotonergic projections	From brainstem raphe nuclei
11. Noradrenergic projections	From the locus ceruleus
12. Orexin projections	From hypothalamus

Table 7.4 Frontal mesoscale networks – intrinsic connectivity networks (ICNs)

Limbic network (SAN)
Salience (ventral attention) network
Executive control network

EI emotional intelligence, *TOM* theory of mind, *SAN* semantic appraisal network, *PMC* presupplementary area, *SMA* supplementary motor area

(Table 7.3). Frontal cognitive processes are not contained in any restricted area or unit and are not modular but rather represented in the connectivity between several large-scale networks (Table 7.4).

Typical brain scan findings are noted in Fig. 7.1.

Overview of Clinical Assessment of PFC Functions

"Frontal network syndromes" is the preferred term rather than frontal lobe syndrome in view of their pan cerebral networking features. Not infrequently, the manifestations of sometimes-profound behavioral disturbance can be missed in the routine, structured office or clinical setting. Real-world situations may be needed to evince these remarkable behavioral deviations, as eloquently demonstrated by Francois Lhermitte [1, 2]. Collateral input is critical as the patient usually does not volunteer behavioral alterations, may dismiss it, or substantiate its normality. Often with FNS, the history carries more weight than the clinical examination. Despite the complexity of functions and assessments, from a clinical perspective, abulia, disinhibition, and executive dysfunction are the key deficits encountered. These correspond to medial PF, orbitofrontal PFC, and lateral PFC. The core physiological frontal systems include the following.

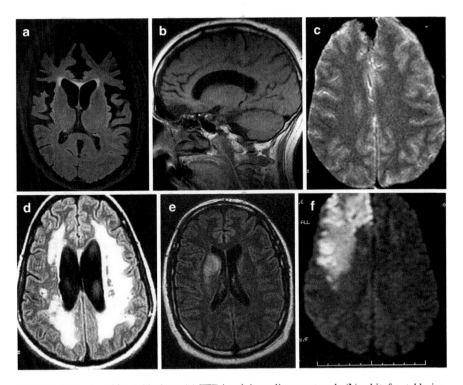

Fig. 7.1 Examples of frontal lesions. (**a**) FTD involving salience network, (**b**) orbitofrontal lesion, (**c**) frontopolar lesion, (**d**) extensive leukoaraiosis involving the frontal subcortical tracts, (**e**) right caudate infarct involving the frontal subcortical tracts, and (**f**) extensive right frontal stroke involving the ECN

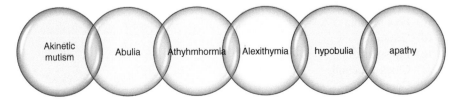

Fig. 7.2 Disorders of conation: abulia spectrum of disorders. Athymhormia absence of voluntary motion, no motor deficit, mental void, and reduced emotional concern. Alexithymia – unable to identify and describe their emotions

Medial PFC

Impairments present with various degrees of abulia, loss of drive, conation, or energization. These range from akinetic mutism to degrees of abulia and apathy (Fig. 7.2). Misdiagnosis may occur with labels such as depression, fatigue, or amotivational syndrome that is not infrequent (Table 7.5). The causative lesions may involve the medial PFC, its associated subcortical circuitry, or adjacent white matter tracts. In addition to

Table 7.5 Conation and initiation disorders: apathy/abulia spectrum, hyperfunction, and subcategories

Decreased
Akinetic mutism
Abulia
Alexithymia
Hypobulia
Apathy
Increased
Akasthisia
ADH/ADHD spectrum
Mania and hypomania
Organic drivenness [3]

the clinical abulia spectrum of disorders, a wide variety of stereotyped and ritualistic behaviors are common and seen in the majority of patients with significant abulia.

Other Behaviors, Stereotypical, Ritualistic

1. Episodic dysmemory due to inattention
2. Impaired registration and impaired retrieval
3. Self-neglect
4. Emotional blunting or flatness
5. Lack of empathy
6. Loss of creativity, initiative, curiosity
7. Stereotyped behavior and ritualistic behavior

    (a) Humming
    (b) Hand rubbing
    (c) Foot tapping
    (d) Grunting
    (e) Lip smacking
    (f) Clock watching
    (g) Counting
    (h) Feasting the same foods

Orbitofrontal Cortex

Lesions here cause principally disinhibition, altered social cognition, and emotional dysregulation.

A wide variety of disinhibition-related behaviors including mirror neuro system disruption or disinhibition may manifest under a manifold of differing presentations that are sometimes difficult to make sense of Table 7.6.

Table 7.6 Disinhibition-related behaviors

1. Socially inappropriate behavior
2. Impulsivity
3. Puerile, profane, facetious, grandiose
4. Irascible and anger attacks
5. Erosion of foresight, insight, or judgment
6. Lose ability to delay gratitude
7. Lose capacity for remorse
8. Abnormal eating behaviors
9. Irritability
10. Aggression, irascible
11. Impairment of comportment
12. Inappropriate social behavior
13. Loss of empathy
14. Emotional dyscontrol (IEED)
15. Excessive jocularity
16. Irresponsible behavior
17. Restlessness
18. Hyperactivity
19. Hypersexuality
20. Hyperorality
21. Incontinence
22. Field-dependent behaviors
(a) More elementary forms
Imitation behavior
Utilization behavior
Echolalia
Environmental dependency syndrome
(b) More complex forms
Forced hyperphasia
Oral spelling behavior
Command-automatism and echopraxia to television
Response to next patient stimulation
Echoplasia

For more detail, see reference [4]

Lateral PFC Functions

The principal deficits include a working memory impairment, a lateral PFC function, also important for white matter (WM), and deficits in task setting (left Dorsolateral prefrontal cortex (DLPFC) function) and monitoring (right DLPFC function). In addition to the bedside tests used in the Coconuts, several other executive function tests can be employed:

1. Alternating sequence task (square and triangle repeated across the page) regarded as a written equivalent of Luria's motor sequence test.

2. Triple loop test (horizontal vs vertical), tests especially for monitoring errors but also TS.
3. Abbreviated Trail Making Test (1A to 5 E) is most often used as an executive function test. Trail A or Comprehensive Trail Making Test (CTMT) 1 and 2 are sensitive to energization functions (recorded as motor and visual search speed) in addition to attention and scanning. Part B or Trails CTMT 5 samples task setting, mental set shifting, and error monitoring. Both DLPFC and medial PFC are therefore evaluated.
4. Abstraction tests evaluate executive function but are prone to cultural differences and influences. With abnormalities, a concreteness emerges that is applicable to both similarities and differences. Typical examples include what category do these belong to; spoon and fork (utensils) as opposed to asking how are these to items alike?
5. Language evaluation is part of the ventral PFC. A frontal speech pattern of Luria may be present with both grammar and syntax intact but relatively confused content. This has been termed the dynamic aphasia of Luria. This represents a selective impairment of verbal planning involving inner speech or endophasia.

Frontal Pole Dysfunctions

The frontopolar cortex integrates information from all of the other prefrontal regions, enabling self-awareness and being aware of one's own state of mind and that of others termed theory of mind (TOM). Together, these functions are termed metacognition. Because of the contiguity of BA 10, 11, and 12, patients with frontopolar (FP) lesions frequently also have orbitofrontal cortex (OFC) lesions that also manifest with behavioral and emotional dysregulations. Bedside testing may include simple questioning such as inquiring whether the person demonstrates sympathy – ability to generate emotion in reaction to another's emotional state or empathy and ability to recognize other's emotional states. TOM can be fractionated into cognitive TOM (deciphering what others think), affective TOM (perceiving what others feel), and conative TOM (being able to influence another person's mental state).

Ventrolateral PFC Functions

Language

Motor language disorders include Broca's aphasia (left hemisphere)
Expressive aprosodia (right hemisphere)
Transcortical motor aphasia
Aphemia – non-fluent speech and normal comprehension and writing, with initial muteness
Central aphasia

Network Presentations

Within the association cortices, each distributed network comprises frontal tempo-ral, parietal, and cingulate cortical components. The networks are also closely inter-twined and interconnected. This arrangement conforms to a multiple parallel processing arrangement with networks interdigitated with each other so that each of the cerebral lobes, for example, may contain several large-scale networks [5]. Large-scale cerebral networks are specifically targeted in a variety of neurodegen-erative diseases as well as TBI, depression, and schizophrenia. Functional imaging has shown impaired functional connectivity in the default mode network (DMN) with AD and in SN in frontotemporal degenerations (FTD).

Semantic Appraisal Network

The semantic valuation and appraisal network (SAN) also termed limbic or preju-dice network is affected in conditions such as PPA semantic variant, presenting with loss of semantic knowledge and significant interpersonal behavior features. The anatomical components of the SAN are detailed in Fig. 7.3. In brief, the SAN com-prises the following:

1. Ventromedial PFC/subgenual cingulate
2. Anterior temporal lobe
3. Basolateral and central amygdala
4. Ventral striatum (caudate)

As a major frontal cortico-limbic network, it functions in the complex socioemo-tional evaluation.

Because of its role in prejudice and stereotyping behavioral assessments, Amodio assigned the label of prejudice network [6]. The SAN interacts with the SN in

Fig. 7.3 Semantic appraisal network hubs (medial view of the brain)

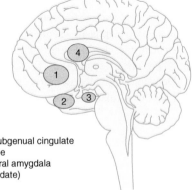

1. Ventromedial PFC/subgenual cingulate
2. Anterior temporal lobe
3. Basolateral and central amygdala
4. Ventral striatum (caudate)

socioemotional evaluations. Other dysfunctions reported with the SAN (SGC node) include mood disorders, mania, and depression. Hodological effects of becoming obsessive at times about other interests such as writing, painting, exercising, or collectionism may emanate [7].

Salience Network Syndromes

The salience network (SN) comprises the principal anatomical components (dorsal anterior cingulate gyrus, amygdala, ventral tegmental area, substantia nigra, fronto-insular). The unique spindle cells or von Economo neurons (VEN) are found in the anterior insula (AI) and anterior cingulate cortex (ACC) that project extensively to other cerebral regions, both hubs of the SN. These facilitate swift communication particularly for the coordinating social dynamics and responses in need of expeditious adaptability. VEN cells in ACC and AI hubs are regarded as an evolutionary response for the high-speed communication between these and the rest of the brain for immediate coordination of activities in a temporal domain. SN activity may also induce a transition between the ECN and DMN. Degeneration of the salience network is implicated in frontotemporal dementias and a spectrum of disorders (Fig. 7.4) with the hypo- and hyperactivation of the networks resulting in specific syndromes (Fig. 7.5). Other networks and structures that are also involved include the following:

- Frontotemporal degenerations and syndromes
- Semantic appraisal network
- Uncinate faciculus
- Orbitofrontal cortex
- Insula
- Temporal pole

This frontotemporal syndrome cluster may present with manifold frontal lobe and frontal network disturbances as well as remote deactivation-type lesions related to diaschisis phenomena.

1. Behavioral variant frontotemporal degeneration (bvFTD) (right hemisphere)
2. Progressive aphasia – semantic and non-fluent aphasia variants (left hemisphere)
3. Gastaut-Geschwind syndrome
4. Klüver–Bucy syndrome
5. Delusional misidentification syndromes
6. Diaschisis-related release phenomena (artistry, literary, architectural)

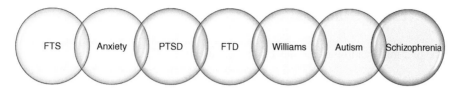

Fig. 7.4 Spectrum of salience network syndromes

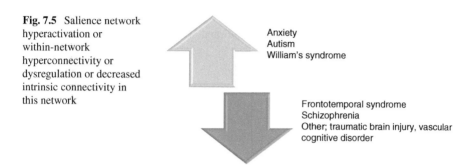

Fig. 7.5 Salience network hyperactivation or within-network hyperconnectivity or dysregulation or decreased intrinsic connectivity in this network

Anxiety
Autism
William's syndrome

Frontotemporal syndrome
Schizophrenia
Other; traumatic brain injury, vascular cognitive disorder

The bvFTD syndrome (RH) presents with a cluster of abnormalities embodied in the international diagnostic criteria of the Daphne criteria. In brief, these include disinhibition, apathy, loss of empathy, perseverations, hyperorality, and neglect [8].

Uncinate Fasciculus Syndromes

The literature refers to three principal functions of the uncinate fasciculus:

- Associative and episodic memory functions
- Linguistic functions
- Socioemotional functions

Insula Syndromes

The literature refers to three principal functions of the uncinate fasciculus:

- Cognitive impairments
- Olfactory, gustatory impairments
- Socioemotional impairments

Klüver Bucy Syndrome

The first four syndromes are most important diagnostically:

- Visual agnosia
- Hypersexuality – homosexuality, heterosexuality, autosexuality
- Hyperorality or "oral" tendency
- Placidity
- Prosopagnosia – loss of people recognition (right temporal lobe)
- Hypermetamorphosis
- Changes in dietary habits – anorexia, bulimia, Gourmand syndrome
- Seizures
- Memory loss

Temporal Pole Lesions [9]

In brief, the TP incorporates highly processed sensory data (dorsal auditory, ventral visual, and medial olfactory and ventral visual radiations) with emotional output. The principal functions are related to the following:

- Socioemotional processing
- Theory of mind
- Face recognition with prosopagnosia if impaired

Orbitofrontal Cortex

The OFC receives inputs from all sensory modalities, including olfactory, gustatory, auditory, visual and somatosensory regions as well as indirectly from all visceral systems. All these are relayed through the thalamus and then to the OFC. With impairments the syndromes that may emerge include the following:

- Inability to differentiate between rewarding and non-rewarding situations
- Inability to alter behavior appropriately when reinforcements change (continuing to respond to stimuli that are no longer rewarded)
- Irresponsibility, lack of affect, and apathy are common
  Impaired interpretation of facial and vocal expressions

Executive Control Network

The frontoparietal executive control network (ECN) comprises bilateral DLPFC, ventrolateral PFC, dorsomedial PFC, lateral parietal, left fronto-insula, caudate, and anterior thalamus (Fig. 7.6). There is also a close reciprocal interaction between the

ECN and SN. The function of the SN in this regard is to modulate between the two networks by balancing allocation of attentional balance in relation to both internal and external sources. These network dynamics involve both complex attention and cognitive control and are an example of overall increased network efficiency. A recent study of video gamers underscored this association and suggested a role for cognitive enhancement [10].

Motor and Sensorimotor Networks

There exists a hierarchy of the various frontal lobe functions, with the frontopolar cortex at the apex of human cognition and behavior and also monitors internal sources of information. The DLPFC primarily monitors and responds to external sources of information and the VPFC holds limited information on line (Fig. 7.7). The capacity for voluntary action is contained in a series of brain networks that include the pre-supplementary motor area (pre-SMA), the anterior PFC, and the parietal areas. Together, these regions and their networks provide information for impending actions, as well as mediating the conscious experience of the intention to act, what specific action to engage in, when to act, and finally in controlling the act. Transforming thoughts into actions is a function of the pre-supplementary motor area (pre-SMA), which is located between the PFC and motor areas, the SMA, and the primary motor cortex BA 4. This has been supported by electrode stimulation of the pre-SMA areas after which patients reported the feeling of a "conscious urge to move." In addition, human transcranial magnetic stimulation (TMS) supports the premise that a function of the pre-SMA is in preparation of movement sequences. Another function of the pre-SMA is in suppressing automatic responses triggered by various environmental stimuli. Lesion studies of the pre-SMA and SMA have been correlated with a hyper-responsiveness including the following:

Fig. 7.6 The executive control network hubs (lateral view of brain)

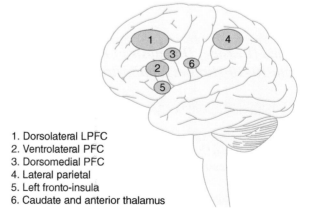

1. Dorsolateral LPFC
2. Ventrolateral PFC
3. Dorsomedial PFC
4. Lateral parietal
5. Left fronto-insula
6. Caudate and anterior thalamus

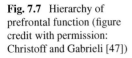
Fig. 7.7 Hierarchy of prefrontal function (figure credit with permission: Christoff and Gabrieli [47])

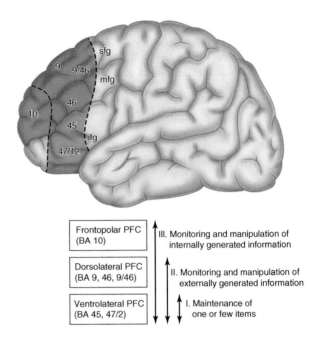

- Field-dependent behavior such as utilization behavior (compulsive urge to grasp items in the contiguous environment (see Table 7.6 for a wide range of various field-dependent behaviors)
- Anarchic hand syndrome: One hand behaves automatically to stimuli and may interfere with the action of the other [11]

From an evolutionary perspective, these motor circuits were associated with innovative behavior that had survival advantages in terms of exploitation and exploration of new resources. In addition, the prefrontal ventromedial cortex coded for possible expected rewards in such endeavors, and the frontopolar regions were the areas engaged in initiating certain exploratory choices [12] (Fig. 7.8).

Rapid (Bedside) Diagnosis of Frontal Networks with 10–30 Minutes Administration Time

The following can all be used depending on the clinical presentation, urgency, and context.

- The Montreal Cognitive Assessment (MOCA)
- Frontal Assessment Battery (FAB)
- Comprehensive cognitive neurological test in stroke (Coconuts)
- Executive Interview Bedside Test (EXIT)

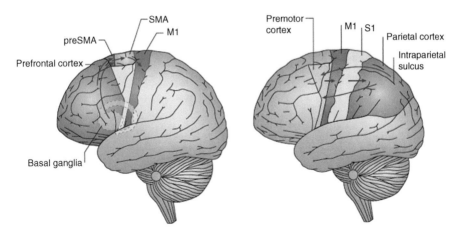

Fig. 7.8 Basal ganglia pre-SMA, SMA circuit (L), parietal premotor circuit (R). (Figure credit: Haggard [48])

Metric Tests

Global Tests

1. Delis Kaplan Executive Function System (DKEF) [13]
2. Wechsler Adult Intelligence Scale (WAIS-IV) components [14]

Clinical Syndrome-Orientated, Questionnaire-Based Tests

3. Frontal Systems Behavior Scale (FRSBE) [15]
4. Behavior Rating Inventory of Executive Function (BRIEF) [16]
5. Frontal Behavioral Inventory (FBI) [17]

Working Memory/Executive Function Tests

6. Trail Making Tests (Comprehensive, Trails A and B, Color Trails) [18]
7. Letter and category fluency list generation [19]
8. Wisconsin Card Sorting Test [20]
9. Tower of London Test [21]
10. Working memory tests (verbal and non-verbal)

Emotional Intelligence Tests

11. Emotional Intelligence Quotient (EQ) – Baron [22]
12. Mayer-Salovey-Caruso Emotional Intelligence Test (MSCEIT) [23]

Tests of Disinhibition/Inhibition

13. Stroop Neuropsychological Screening Test [24]
14. Iowa Gambling Test [25]

Autism

15. Autism Diagnostic Interview – Revised [26]
16. Autism Spectrum Quotient [27]

ADHD

17. Brown Attention Deficit Disorder Scales [28]

Depression

18. CES-D (Center for Epidemiological Studies Depression Scale) [29]
19. Beck Depression Scale [30]
20. Hamilton Depression Inventory [31]

Behavioral Neurological Tests

21. Faux Pas Test [32]
22. Reading the Mind in the Eyes Test [33]
23. Hotel Task [34]
24. Multiple Errands Test [35]
25. Ambiguous Figures Test [36]

Creativity Tests

26. Torrance Test of Creative Thinking [37]

Other Tests That Predominantly Assess Frontal Network Systems

27. Visual Search and Attention Test [38]
28. Rey Complex Figure Test [39]

Clinical Tests: Qualitative Without Normative Data

29. The Executive Control Battery [40]

A Novel Approach

30. The metacognitive battery incorporating neurological, neuropsychological, and neuropsychiatric syndromes [41]

Aphasia Tests Useful in Motor Aphasia, Dysnomia, and Aphasias in General

31. Western Aphasia Battery [42]
32. Boston Diagnostic Aphasia Evaluation [43]

Elementary Neurological

Clinical neurological assessment of:

Olfaction (The Smell Identification Test, Sensonics [44])
Gait (modified Gait Abnormality Rating Scale) [45]
Incontinence
Primitive reflexes (grasp reflex, palmo-mental reflex, sucking reflex)
Volitional eye movements [46]

References

1. Lhermitte F, Pillon B, Seradura M. Human autonomy and the frontal lobes. Part 1: imitation and utilization behavior. A neuropsychological study of 75 patients. Ann Neurol. 1986;19:326–34.
2. Lhermitte F. Human autonomy and the frontal lobes. Part II: patient behavior in complex and social situations: the "environmental dependency syndrome". Ann Neurol. 1986;19:335–43.
3. Kahn E. Psychopathic personalities. New Haven: Yale University Press; 1931.
4. Hoffmann M. Cognitive, conative and Behavioral neurology. New York: Springer; 2016.
5. Yeo BTT, Kriene FM, Sepulcre J, et al. The organization of the human cerebral cortex estimated by intrinsic functional connectivity. J Neurophysiol. 2011;106:1125–65.
6. Fourie MM, Thomas KG, Amodio DM, et al. Neural correlates of experienced moral emotion: an fMRI investigation of emotion in response to prejudice feedback. Soc Neurosci. 2014;9:203–18.
7. Wu TQ, Miller ZA, Adhimoolam B, et al. Verbal creativity in semantic variant primary progressive aphasia. Neurocase. 2015;21:73–8.

8. Boutoleau-Bretonnière C, Evrard C, Benoît Hardouin J, et al. DAPHNE: a new tool for the assessment of the Behavioral variant of Frontotemporal dementia. Dement Geriatr Cogn Disord Extra. 2015;5:503–16.

9. Olsen IR, Plotzker A, Ezzyat Y. The enigmatic temporal pole: a review of findings on social and emotional processing. Brain. 2007;130:1718–31.

10. Gong D, et al. Functional integration between salience and central executive networks. A role for action video game experience. Neural Plast. 2016; 9803165

11. Fried I, et al. Functional organization of human supplementary motor cortex studied by electrical stimulation. J Neurosci. 1991;11:3656–66.

12. Daw ND, et al. Cortical substrates for exploratory decisions in humans. Nature. 2006;441:876–9.

13. Delis DC, Kaplan E, Kramer JH. DKEFS. The Psychological Corporation. London, UK: Harcourt Assessment Company; 2001.

14. Wechsler D. Wechsler adult intelligence scale. 4th ed. San Antonio: The Psychological Corporation. Harcourt Brace and Company; 2008.

15. Grace J, Malloy PF. Frontal systems behavior scale. Lutz: PAR Neuropsychological Assessment Resources Inc; 2001.

16. Roth RM, Isquith PK, Gioia GA. BRIEF-A. Behavior rating inventory of executive function-adult version. Lutz: PAR Neuropsychological Assessment Resources Inc; 2005.

17. Kertesz A, Davidson W, Fox H. Frontal behavioural inventory: diagnostic criteria for frontal lobe dementia. Can J Neurol Sci. 1997;24:29–36.

18. Reynolds CR. Comprehensive trail making test. Austin: Pro-Ed; 2002.

19. Gladsjo JA, Walden Miller W, Heaton RK. Norms for letter and category fluency: demographic corrections for age, education and ethnicity. Lutz: Psychological Assessment Resources Inc; 1999.

20. Heaton RK. Wisconsin card sorting test computer version 4. Lutz: PAR Psychological Assessment Resources; 2003.

21. Culbertson WC, Zillmer EA. Tower of London. Toronto: Multi Health Systems Inc; 2001.

22. Bar-On R. The Bar-On Emotional Quotient Inventory (EQ-i): Technical manual. Toronto, Canada: Multi-Health Systems; 1997.

23. MSCEIT. Mayer, Salovey, & Caruso. Toronto: Multi Health Systems Inc; 2002.

24. Trenerry MR, Crosson B, DeBoe J, Leber WR. Stroop neuropsychological screening test. Lutz: Psychological Assessment Resources (PAR); 1989.

25. Bechara A. Iowa Gambling Test. Lutz: Psychological Assessment Resources Inc; 2007.

26. Rutter M, Le Couteur A, Lord C. ADI-R. Los Angeles: Western Psychological Services; 2005.

27. Baron-Cohen S, Wheelwright S, Skinner R, Martin J, Clubley E. The autism Spectrum quotient (AQ): evidence from Asperger syndrome/high-functioning autism, males and females, scientists and mathematicians. J Autism Dev Disord. 2001;31:5–17.

28. Brown TE. Brown attention deficit disorder scales. Hamden: The Psychological Corporation. A Harcourt Assessment Company; 1996.

29. Radloff L. The CES-D scale: a self report depression scale for research in the general population. Appl Psychol Meas. 1977;1(3):385–401.

30. Beck AT, Steer RA, Brown GK. Beck depression inventory II. San Antonio: Psychological Corporation; 1996.

31. Reynolds WM, Kobak KA. Hamilton depression inventory. Lutz: Psychological Assessment Resources Inc; 1995.

32. Stone VE, Baron-Cohen S, Knight RT. Frontal lobe contribution to theory of mind. J Cogn Neurosci. 1998;10:640–56.

33. Baron-Cohen S, Joliffe T, Mortimore C, Robertson M. Another advanced test of theory of mind: evidence from very high functioning adults with autism or Asperger syndrome. J Child Psychol Psychiatry. 1997;38:813–22.

34. Manly T, Hawkins K, Evans J, Woldt K, Robertson IH. Rehabilitation of executive function: facilitation of effective goal management on complex tasks using periodic auditory alerts. Neuropsychologia. 2002;40:271–81.

35. Knight C, Alderman N, Burgess PW. Development of a simplified version of the multiple errrands test for use in hospital settings. Neuropsychol Rehabil. 2002;12:231–55.

36. Windmann S, Wehrmann M, Calabrese P, Guntuerken O. Role of the prefrontal cortex in attentional control over bistable vision. J Cogn Neurosci. 2006;18:456–71.

37. Torrance EP. Influence of dyadic interaction on creative functioning. Psychol Rep. 1970;26:391–4.

38. Trenerry MR, Cross B, De Boe J, Leber WR. Visual search and attention test (VSAT). Lutz: Psychological Assessment Resources Inc; 1990.

39. Holmes Bernstein J, Waber DP. Developmental scoring system for the Rey Osterrieth complex figure. Lutz: Psychological Assessment Resources Inc; 1996.

40. Goldberg E, Podelle K, Bilder R, Jaeger J. The executive control battery. Melbourne: Psych Press; 1999.

41. Hoffmann M, Schmitt F. Metacognition in stroke: bedside assessment and relation to location, size and stroke severity. Cogn Behav Neurol. 2006;19(2):85–94.

42. Kertesz A. The western aphasia battery. The Psychological Corporation. London, UK: Harcourt Brace Jovanovich Inc.; 1982.

43. Goodglass H, Kaplan E, Barresi B. Boston diagnostic aphasia test. 3rd ed. Philadelphia: Lippincott, Williams, Wilkins; 2001.

44. Doty R. Sensonics Inc. Haddon Heights NJ, USA, 2006. www.sensonics.com.

45. Van Swearingham M, Paschal KA, Bonino P, Yang J-F. The modified gait abnormality rating scale for recognizing the risk of recurrent falls in community dwelling elderly adults. Phys Ther. 1996;76:994–1002.

46. Jong's D. The neurologic examination. Philadephia: Lipincott Williams and Wilkins; 2005.

47. Christoff K, Gabrieli JDE. The frontopolar cortex and human cognition: evidence for a rostrocaudal hierarchical organization within the human prefrontal cortex. Psychobiology. 2000;28:168–86.

48. Haggard P. Human volition: towards a neuroscience of will. Nat Rev Neurosci. 2008;9:934–6.

Chapter 8
Default Mode Network (Mentalizing) and Limbic Network for Explicit Episodic Memory Syndromes

In addition to clinical testing indicating a significant memory loss, brain scan lesions that implicate memory impairment are depicted in Fig. 8.1. The default mode network (DMN) may also be referred to as a memory network, as its key function is accessing memory and also creating memories. Major hubs of the DMN intrinsic connectivity network (ICN) are the medial parietal area and medial prefrontal area with other important areas including the lateral parietal, lateral temporal cortical areas, and posterior cingulate precuneus. On functional imaging, these regions show greatest activity during the resting mode (Fig. 8.2). The precuneus region on its own consumes more than 35% of glucose, more than any other cortical region – hence the term "hot spots." Furthermore, the precuneus and contiguous posteromedial cortical regions display marked deactivation in a number of cerebral pathophysiological conditions including the following.

- General anesthesia
- Slow wave sleep
- Hypnotic states
- Vegetative state
- Minimally conscious states
- Temporal loss of self-awareness (epilepsy, schizophrenia)

This precuneus activity may be an important marker for minimally conscious states (MCS) as the precuneus hypoactivity is the initial area that improves and has been corroborated with clinical improvement. The DMN subserves several key memory-related processes including other roles:

1. Episodic encoding
2. Retrieval
3. Autobiographical
4. Metamemory processes including mental time travel
5. Socioemotional processing and theory of mind (TOM)
6. Moral decision-making

© Springer Nature Switzerland AG 2020
M. Hoffmann, *Clinical Mentation Evaluation*,
https://doi.org/10.1007/978-3-030-46324-3_8

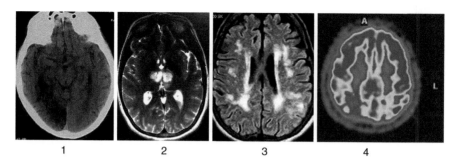

Fig. 8.1 Right posterior cerebral and medial temporal lobe infarcts (1), bilateral thalamic infarcts (tegmentothalamic syndrome) (2), extensive leukoaraiosis (3), and occipital PET scan hypometabolism in occipital cortical atrophy (Benson's syndrome) variant of Alzheimer's disease (4)

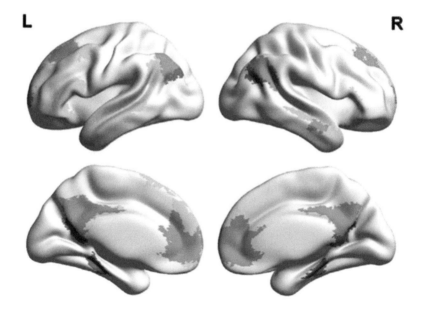

Fig. 8.2 Default Mode Network Core subsystem (orange) and MTL (red) and dm-PFC (yellow) subsystems. The dm-PFC subsystem is involved with metacognition such as with mentalizing or reflecting upon the present time with respect to one's self or others. The MTL subsystem is preferentially engaged when making episodic or contextual retrieval of information or when simulating the future [1]

The brain has intrinsic processing power, with a large proportion of the resting activity (estimated at 60–80% of all energy used by the brain), occurring in circuitry unrelated to any external event. It has also been estimated that performing a specific task consumes only ~5% of underlying baseline activity. DMN activity may underlie common, everyday mental errors and also implicated in complex clinical disorders such as depression, schizophrenia, autism, and Alzheimer's disease. The topographic distribution of the default mode network components mirrors closely that of fibrillar amyloid deposition in AD patients as measured by amyloid PET scans. The beta-amyloid accumulation as assessed by the imaging MRI based modality using Pittsburgh Compound B (PIB) correspond to the synaptic dysfunction that is assessed by FDG-PET brain scanning which in turn follows neuronal loss as assessed by volumetric MRI studies. These processes can all be documented prior to dementia onset. Hence, AD may be characterized as a DMN-related disease process [2]. Petrella et al. reported lower connectivity in the default mode network in people diagnosed with mild cognitive impairment (MCI) as well as those with MCI who subsequently developed AD within a 2–3 year period [3]. Another study by Seeley et al. documented five different neurodegenerative syndromes corresponding to five different ICNs [4].

The DMN has influence with the other ICNs for the purposes of coordinating activity among many diverse brain regions. This allows many cerebral regions to act in concert when presented with stimuli or tasks. This has been compared to the conductor of a symphony orchestra and termed "The Brain's Orchestral Conductor." Slow cortical potentials that can be detected by functional MRI scanning with a cycle frequency of 1/10 s are proposed as the equivalent of the "conductors baton" [5]. There are particularly close interactions and connections with the DMN, frontoparietal network (FPN), and executive control network (ECN) [6].

Memory classification: A Neurobiological and Clinical System Approach

The clinically appreciated disorders can be categorized into the following:

Temporal based alteration

- Anterograde and retrograde amnesia
- Short-term, long–term, and prospective memories

Hypo- and hyperfunction

- Amnesia
- Hyperthymesia (Savant syndromes)

Neuroanatomy of Memory Systems

Memory subsystem	Information, type/time	Neuroanatomical components
Working (7 digits forward/5 back)	Seconds to minutes	DLPFC, PPA, TL, subcortex
Episodic (word lists, short story)	Minutes to years	PFC, FPC, MT ATN, F, MB
Semantic (factual information)	Minutes to years	Lateral inferior temporal region

Memory subsystem	Information, type/time	Neuroanatomical components
Procedural (biking, walking)	Minutes to years	SMA, BG, cerebellum

PFC prefrontal cortex, *FPC* frontopolar cortex, *MT* mamillothalmic tract, *ATN* anterior thalamic nucleus, *F* fornix, *MB* mamillary bodies, *DLPFC* dorsolateral prefrontal cortex, *PPA* posterior parietal areas, *TL* temporal lobe, *PHR* parahippocampal region, *SMA* supplementary motor area, *BG* basal ganglia

Clinical Categories

- Episodic memory (visual, verbal)
- Working memory (visuospatial)
- Semantic
- Procedural
- Metamemory

Episodic Memory

Episodic memory allows us to travel back in time and forward in time. Episodic memory is an autobiographical association with past experiences and mental time travel into the future. The neurophysiology of the stages in forming new memories involve the following processes and networks:

- Episodic memory formation and transfer from short- to long-term memory requires medial temporal lobe activation which plays a central role in episodic memory retention.
- New information encoding requires participation of the executive control and semantic processing networks (temporal poles, lateral temporal lobes).
- The Papez circuit structures are important in long-term memory formation.

Fig. 8.3 Schematic diagram of the principal episodic memory components: frontal, basal forebrain, amygdala, thalamus, and medial parietal

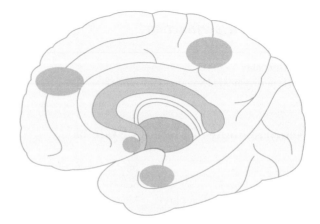

- The retrieval process requires increased activity in the principal hubs and networks subserving executive control, default mode networks, as well as the posterior cingulate and precuneus brain areas (Fig. 8.3).

Working Memory

Working memory is the cognitive ability to maintain information online for brief periods of time, which is measured in seconds to minutes, and is the processing information which allows us to construct sentences, work with numbers, for example, calculations, as well as thoughts and actions. This is often referred to as "short-term memory." Working memory is measured in seconds to minutes and episodic memory is measured in minutes (short-term episodic memory) to years (long-term episodic memory). Working memory may be conceived of as a kind of operating system of the brain and underlies the core frontal processes such as disinhibition, attention, and initiation – the most fundamental and cardinal functions of the frontal lobes. The principal working memory hubs include the following:

1. Epoptic process: Mid-dorsolateral prefrontal cortex monitors information
2. Manipulation of information: Posterior parietal region around the intraparietal sulcus (Fig. 8.4)
3. Both regions interact with the superior temporal region for sensory information (auditory, visual verbal, multimodal)
4. The principal fiber tract's sub-serving working memory include the following:

   (a) Superior longitudinal fasciculus
   (b) Middle longitudinal fasciculus
   (c) Extreme capsule

Fig. 8.4 Schematic diagrams of the major hubs of working memory: frontal, parietal (purple), semantic memory; inferotemporal, anterior temporal lobe (blue), and procedural memory; supplementary motor area, basal ganglia, cerebellum (green)

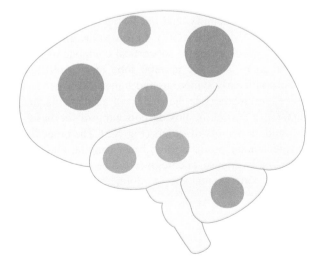

Semantic Memory

Semantic memory refers to the knowledge we possess about the world and people in general, as well as specific terms relating to facts about objects, people, animal and historical events. Episodic memory is concerned with the retrieval of facts and semantic memory is concerned with the knowledge of facts and does not have a so called autobiographical "tag". The autobiographic "tag" is also termed autonoesis, and refers to the linking of memories in either in a time based (temporal) or spatial capacity. Semantic memory impairments generally present with naming difficulty. The neurobiology of semantic memory involves distributed hubs in the bilateral inferolateral cortices (Fig. 8.4). The left DLPFC encodes episodic memories and the right DLPFC is concerned with the retrieval of episodic memories. Semantic memory retrieval is a function of the left inferotemporal lobe hemisphere. Facial recognition is a semantic memory function based in the right anterior temporal lobe amenable to testing with the Famous Faces Test [7]. During childhood development, a progressive formation of episodic memories occurs which eventually becomes semantic memory traces. An initial learning process of learning how to use a tool, implement, or device begins as an episodic memory experience and later becomes long-term memory and semantic memory or factual information. Hence, semantic memory is initially derived from episodic memory experiences.

Procedural Memory

This refers to knowing how to perform or do something, without there being specific awareness for the task at hand including playing a musical instrument, driving a car, bicycle riding, typing shoelaces, and reading. These automatic abilities operate at the non-conscious level and are subtypes of long-term memory and an implicit-type memory, and are learned through repetitive activity. In sport, the concept of "muscle memory" refers to the gradual shift from prefrontal cortical circuitry involvement to subcortical components (basal ganglia), supplementary motor areas, superior parietal lobe and cerebellum with protracted training. People with early symptoms and signs of Parkinson's disease show impairment of procedural memory in the context of normal episodic memory function. Strokes, tumors, or carbon monoxide poisoning of the basal ganglia similarly produces procedural memory disorders (Fig. 8.5). The procedural memory hubs include the supplementary motor cortex, basal ganglia, and cerebellum. Collateral inquiry from family, spouse, or caregiver will be informative regarding impaired ability to perform certain mundane or routine tasks that they had been able to perform flawlessly.

Fig. 8.5 Bilateral
hyperintensities in the
basal nuclei consequent to
carbon monoxide exposure

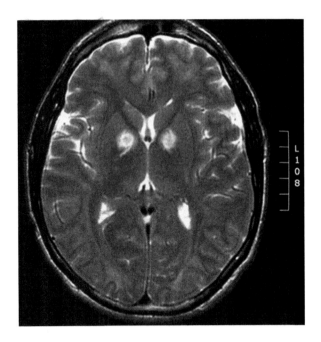

Metamemory

This refers to the concept of "self-knowledge," or having insight into one's own memory abilities or capabilities as well as the accuracy of both retrospective and prospective performance judgments.

Bedside Memory Evaluation

First screen for attention, alertness, language, and normal vision

1. *Working memory (immediate memory)*

    (a) Digit span – normal is 7 forward and 5 backward
    (b) Serial 7's (can use serial 3's to make it simpler)
    (c) Reciting months of year in reverse order

2. *Episodic memory (short- and long-term memories)*

    (a) Verbal – words (3–10), recite after 10 min or more
    (b) Visual – geometric shapes
    (c) Story recall

Fig. 8.6 Three Words
Three Shapes Test.
Weintraub [21]

  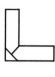

PRIDE   HUNGER   STATION

(d) Three Words Three Shapes Test: Allows testing of (i) verbal, non-verbal, (ii) incidental recall (copy and WM), (iii) effortful encoding (present items 3 times more until score ≥5), (iv) delayed recall (after 10–15 min), and (v) recognition (retention function) – list of several words and shapes presented including original items (Fig. 8.6)

(e) Remote memory – Recite last 3 presidents or 3 important personal dates (graduations)

3. *Semantic memory*

(a) Boston Naming Test
(b) Semantic fluency – animal naming
(c) Vocabulary Test
(d) NW University Famous Faces Test

4. *Procedural memory (previous implicit non-declarative memory)*

(a) Use parts of words or drawings and guess possible words or items that may be generated. What word, for example, RA--I-, PL--B--, S-F-T- which could generate RAISIN, PLUMBER, SAFETY

5. *Metamemory*
This may be evaluated by the feeling of knowing (FOK) and judgment of learning (JOL) tests [8, 9].

Metric/Quantitative Memory Evaluation [10]

- *Rey Auditory Verbal Learning Test*

  – A 15-word category A list followed by a 15-word interference category B list, followed by two post-list B interference recall trials – immediate and delayed – then a recognition trial with distractor words [11]

- *Wechsler Memory Scale IV* [12].

  – Probably the most widely used memory test, which is a comprehensive battery that deciphers memory and learning according to the domains of working and episodic memories into both visual and verbal components as well as recall and recognition scores for both

- *California Verbal Learning Test version II (CVLT-II)*

  – The CVLT II is now available as both standard and short forms. The CVLT employs both cued recall and recognition formats
  – The CVLT II SF, which has one list of 9 words, 3 categories, and 4 learning trials [13]

- *Hopkins Verbal Learning Test*

  – This test consists of 12 word lists followed by a 24 recognition list and 6 alternate forms [14]

- *Repeatable Battery for the Assessment of Neuropsychological Status (RBANS)*

  – This test includes a short story recall which is considered the most important way of testing day to day memory usage and has a story and a 10-word list test paradigm [15].

- *Remote memory*

  – Famous Faces Test [7]

- *Visual recall*

  – Rey-Osterrieth Complex Figure Test [16]

- *Semantic Memory tests*

  – Boston Naming Test including the cueing option [17]
  – Category fluency for animals is impaired with semantic dysmemory.
  – Pyramids and Palms Test [18]

- *Procedural memory tests*

  – Serial Reaction Time Task
  – Pursuit rotor task – visual motor task that can be accomplished by following a mark on a computer screen in a circular fashion by operating a computer mouse [19, 20].

References

1. Zhou HX, Chen X, Shen YQ et al. Rumination and the default mode network: Meta-analysis of brain imaging studies and implications for depression. Neuroimage 2020;206:116–287.
2. Jagust WJ, Mormino EC. Lifespan brain activity, β-amyloid, and Alzheimer's disease. Trends Cogn Sci. 2011;15(11):520–6. https://doi.org/10.1016/j.tics.2011.09.004.
3. Petrella JR, Sheldon FC, Prince SE, Calhoun VD, Doraiswamy PM. Default mode network connectivity in stable vs progressive mild cognitive impairment. Neurology. 2011;76:511–7.
4. Seeley WW, et al. Neurodegenerative disease target large scale human brain networks. Neuron. 2009;62:42–52.
5. Raichle ME. The brain's dark energy. Sci Am 2010;302(3):44–9.

6. Alcami P, Pereda AE. Beyond plasticity: the dynamic impact of electrical synapses on neural circuits. Nat Rev Neurosci. 2019;20:253–71.
7. Hodges JR, Salmon DP, Butters N. Recognition and naming of famous faces in Alzheimer's disease: a cognitive analysis. Neuropsychologia. 1993;31:775–88.
8. Fleming SM, Dolan RJ. The neural basis of metacognitive ability. Philos Trans R Soc B. 2012;367:1338–49. https://doi.org/10.1098/rstb.2011.0417.
9. Pronin E. Perception and misperception of bias in human judgment. Trends Cogn Sci. 2007;11:37–43.
10. Lezak MD, Howieson DB, Bigler ED, Tranel D. Neuropsychological assessment. 5th ed. Oxford: Oxford University Press; 2012.
11. Rey A. L'examen Clinique en psychologie. Paris: Presses Universitaires de France; 1964.
12. Wechsler D. Wechsler memory scale and Wechsler adult intelligence scale IV technical manual. San Antonio: Psychological Corporation; 2009.
13. Delis DC, Kramer JH, Kaplan E, Ober BA. California verbal learning test. 2nd ed. San Antonio: Texas Psychological Corporation; 2000.
14. Brandt J. The Hopkins verbal learning test: development of a new memory test with six equivalent forms. Clin Neuropsychol. 1991;5:125–42.
15. Randolph C. Manual: repeatable battery for the assessment of neuropsychological status. San Antonio: Psychological Corporation; 1998.
16. Osterrieth PA. Le test de copie d'une figure complexe. Archive de Psychologie 1944;30:206–356; Rey A. L'examen psychologique dans les cas d'encephalopathie traumatique. Arch Psychol 1941;28:286–340.
17. Kaplan E, Goodglass H, Weintraub S. Boston naming test. 2nd ed. Boston: Lippincott Williams & Wilkins; 2001.
18. Howard D, Patterson K. Pyramids and palm trees: a test of semantic access from pictures and words. Bury St Edmunds: Thames Valley Test Company; 1992.
19. Balota DA, Connor LT, Ferraro FR. Implicit memory and the formation of new associations in nondemented Parkinson's disease individuals and individuals with senile dementia of the Alzheimer type: a serial reaction time (SRT) investigation. Brain Cogn. 1993;21:163–80.
20. Bullemer P, Nissen MJ, Willingham DB. On the development of procedural knowledge. J Exp Psychol Learn Mem Cogn. 1989;15:1047–60.
21. Weintraub S, Peavy GM, O'Connor M, et al. Three words three shapes: a clinical test of memory. J Clin Exp Neuropsychol. 2000;22(2):267–78.

Chapter 9
Right Dominant Frontoparietal Network for Spatial Orientation (Dorsal Attention and Visuospatial Attention)

With usually preserved communication, unlike left hemisphere aphasia–related communication impairment, right hemisphere (RH) lesions reveal a manifold of cognitive disorders. Each of these may be the key to monitoring an improvement or deterioration of the clinical status or disease pathophysiology. Furthermore, the RH is dominant for more known entities (at least measurable by us thus far) than the left hemisphere (Table 9.1).

In brief, right hemisphere function can be conceived as having two principal properties being dominance for both attention and emotion. The disorders listed below are all derivatives of these two major cognitive faculties. Attention requires considerable processing resources and is the cognitive ability that selects stimuli for further evaluation at the same time ignoring others. Christoff Koch had a particularly succinct definition: *"Attention is evolution's answer to information overload. No brain can process all incoming information"* [5].

Table 9.1 Hemisphere dominance [1–4]

Right hemisphere dominance
Attention
Emotion
Prosody
Melody
Spatial construction
Body image
Left hemisphere dominance
Language
Praxis
Calculation/analytical/mathematical
Temporal stimuli sequencing

Right Hemisphere Syndromes

Typical examples of right hemisphere lesions, both stroke and inflammatory lesions, are depicted in Fig. 9.1. Because of the frequent inattention, denial, or neglect components, these syndromes are often termed clinically "silent."

More Common Right Hemisphere Lesion Disorders

Attentional disorders
Neglect syndromes
Anosognosia for hemiparesis
Visuospatial dysfunction
Aprosodia

Attention

The right hemisphere is dominant for both attention and arousal. One of the most common neurological consultations is for evaluation of the acute confusional state (ACS) which reflects a disturbance of the dorsal attentional system, with major network hubs including Dorsolateral prefrontal cortex (DLPFC) posterior parietal and medial temporal brain regions (Fig. 9.2). ACS presents with a global disturbance of the attentional matrix with the principal clinical features including inattention, impaired vigilance, distractibility, and fluctuating cognition impairment (multi-domains but principally working memory). The level of consciousness is

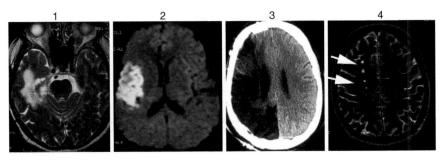

1-Isolated right temporal lobe inflammatory process, 2- right frontoparietal infarct, 3 – large right fronto-parietO- occipital infarct, 4- right ACA-MCA watershed infarct

Fig. 9.1 Right temporal lobe lesions often present with relatively "silent brain lesions." 1, Isolated right temporal lobe inflammatory process; 2, right frontoparietal infarct; 3, large right fronto-parieto-occipital infarct; 4, right ACA-MCA watershed infarct

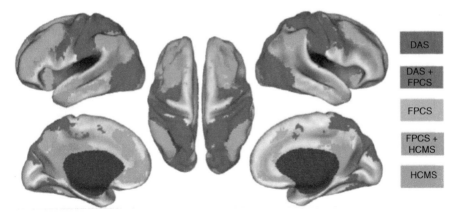

Fig. 9.2 The major intrinsic connectivity networks: dorsal attention system (DAS; blue), fronto-parietal control salience (FPCS; light green), default mode network (DMN; orange) systems. Overlap of salience and DMN (dark green) and DAS and salience (red). (Figure with permission: Vincent et al. [99])

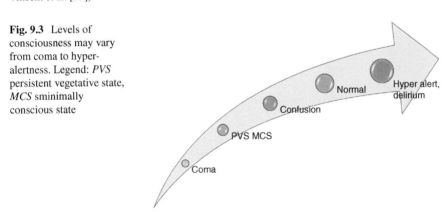

Fig. 9.3 Levels of consciousness may vary from coma to hyper-alertness. Legend: *PVS* persistent vegetative state, *MCS* sminimally conscious state

altered and may vary from coma to hyper-alertness or delirium (either hyperactive or hypoactive delirium) (Fig. 9.3). Hallucinations, delusions, and disorganized thinking may form part of the presentation.

The degree of spatial neglect on the other hand is the clinical presentation of the domain-specific systems impairment, reflective of attention disturbance within the person's extrapersonal space. Hence, neglect is a disorder of spatial attention. The network subserving spatial attention involves the posterior parietal cortex, the cingulate gyrus, frontal eye fields, the subcortical components (thalamus, striatum, superior collicus) and interacts with the ascending reticular activating system (Fig. 9.4). These may be depicted in a three-tier system with the frontal subcortical parietal cortical network referring to the top of the hierarchy and the mid component being represented by the circuitry subserving various sensory modalities and leading to domain-specific or modality-specific deficits such as the neglect syndromes.

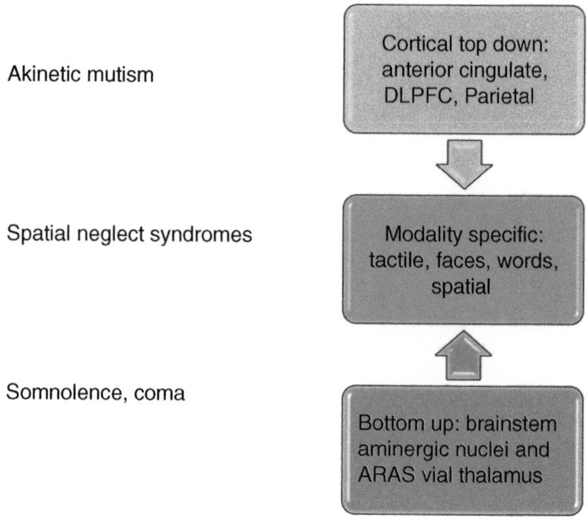

Fig. 9.4 Attentional circuits: top down, bottom up, middle modality specific and clinical examples

Akinetic mutism

Cortical top down: anterior cingulate, DLPFC, Parietal

Spatial neglect syndromes

Modality specific: tactile, faces, words, spatial

Somnolence, coma

Bottom up: brainstem aminergic nuclei and ARAS vial thalamus

The inferior component, the ascending neurotransmitter systems, provides modulation of various kinds, but its key role is arousal [6].

The top-down component of the attentional circuitry may at times cause features of a domain-general or a domain-specific presentation of attention derangement. Lesions of the frontal, posterior parietal, or medial temporal brain regions can produce an ACS.

Bedside Testing

Confusion Assessment Method (CAM): For Diagnosis, Items 1 and 2 and Either 3 or 4 [7] Are Required

1. Acute onset and fluctuating course (from family/nurse)
2. Inattention (forward digit span)
3. Disorganized thinking (rambling, confused conversation)
4. Altered level of consciousness (alert, hyperalert, hypoalert, stupor, coma)

Cobe-20 (Chap. 5)

COBE - 20 (Cognitive and Behavioral Evaluation) described in more detail in Chap. 5.

Visuospatial Function

Although a wide variety of lesion sites in the brain may be associated with visuospatial dysfunction, the right posterior brain areas, specifically the parietal lobe, are particularly involved. Visuospatial function has both sensory (visuoperceptual) and motor components (visuomotor) which can be tested separately as follows:

- Visuoperceptual – test by judgment of line orientation
- Visuomotor or visuoconstructual ability – a variety of simple diagrams may be copied such as copying two-dimensional images of a daisy flower, 3D Necker cube [8], intersecting pentagons, or clock drawing representing an approximate gradation from easy to more difficult tasks.

Metric Testing

- Rey-Osterrieth Complex Figure Test which is scored according to 18 items, each scored 0, 1, or 2 for a maximum of 36, both for copying and after a 15-minute delay [9].
- Taylor Complex Figure, 18 items each, scored 0, 1, or 2 for a maximum of 36 [10].
- Benson Complex Figure Test [11].
- RBANS figure, scored for 20 items [12].

Anosognosia

Most often seen in the first few days to weeks after right hemisphere lesion such as stroke, the patient demonstrates an underestimation or denial of illness or deficit such as hemiplegia. It may vary from a partial denial or gross underestimation of weakness with no acknowledgment of any weakness at all. In the acute stages after RH stroke, these syndromes may affect up to 58–73% of patients [13] that typically resolve relatively rapidly [14–16]. Some patients maintain that the left arm is foreign or representing a stranger lying in their bed and have been reported to attempt throwing the limb out of bed [17].

Clinical evaluation can be performed by simple, rapid bedside scales or semi-quantitative measures depending on what specific deficit denial is present. With anosognosia for hemiparesis, for example, the Bisiach scale may be employed.

Bedside Testing

Bisiach scale [18]:

0 – Deficit spontaneously reported to general questioning
1 – Deficit reported only after specific question about limb strength
2 – Deficit acknowledged after examination demonstrated weakness
3 – Deficit denied even after demonstration of weakness or plegia

Metric Measures: May Be Used for Monitoring or for Research

- The Denial of Illness Scale [19]
- Cutting's Anosognosia Questionnaire [20]
- The Bimanual task of Cocchini [21]
- The Catherine Bergego Scale [22]

Prosody

The right hemisphere is dominant for emotional processing including prosody which refers to the melodic intonation associated with speaking and regarded as an important paralinguistic language component. The motor or expressive aspects of affective prosody can be assessed during the patient interview, by paying attention to the person's intonation whether flat or monotone. Repetition of affective prosody may be evaluated by requesting the person to repeat a sentence in a happy, sad, or angry voice. Prosody comprehension may be evaluated by asking the person to evaluate the examiner's pronunciation of a sentence said in a happy, sad, or angry voice. Testing should be devoid of facial expressions or gestures facilitation, for example, by standing behind the person. An aprosodia classification can therefore be deduced into the following:

1. Sensory aprosodia – there is appropriate affective prosody during speech and gesturing, but the auditory appreciation of affective prosody is impaired. Furthermore, when testing emotional gesturing which is appreciated visually by the person, this is also impaired.
2. Motor or expressive aprosodia – the person has a monotone speech with paucity of spontaneous gesturing. Affective prosody repetition is impaired with normal affective prosody (auditory) comprehension. Emotional gesturing by visual comprehension remains intact.
3. Global aprosodia – there is an overall lack of prosody and gesturing with a flattened affect, impairment of comprehension, and repetition of affective prosody as well as visual comprehension of emotional gesturing [23–26].

A Brief Bedside Prosody Test

Spontaneous Prosody

Does person impart affect into conversation through prosody (1) and gestures (1)?

- Scoring
- Present   2
- Absent   0
- Total /2

Repetition of Affective Prosody

A sentence ("today is a sunny and windy day") devoid of emotional words is said in a

- Happy
- Angry
- Sad

tone of voice by the examiner which, the person repeats in the same affective intonation

- Scoring
- Present   1
- Absent   0
- Total /3

Comprehension of Affective Prosody

The examiner says the sentence ("today is a sunny and windy day"), free of emotional words, in a

- Happy
- Angry
- Sad

tone of voice, whereafter the person needs to identify the emotion.

- Scoring
- Present   1
- Absent   0
- Total /3
- Grand total   /8

Subtypes of the Principal Right Hemisphere Syndromes

Attentional and Neglect Disorders [27–32]

1. Motor neglect – test with line bisection tasks (10 cm long) in the horizontal, vertical, and angular (45 degrees) planes. Cancellation tasks such as shapes, letters, or numbers can also be employed.
2. Sensory neglect – bilateral simultaneous stimulation, with eyes closed can be performed for tactile and touch both forearms at once.
3. Spatial neglect – observed during the instruction to draw items such as a flower, cube, house, or person; such patients may ignore parts of the picture.

4. Egocentric – neglect of their own space or personal space.
5. Allocentric neglect, peripersonal space neglect, extrapersonal or reaching space neglect.
6. Object-centered neglect – target-associated features whereby the left side of targets is relatively neglected.
7. Environment-centered neglect – refers to the relationship between the environment and body and may be revealed by right parietal lesions.
8. Representational neglect – neglect for items recalled from memory and may be conveyed when recalling a scene from memory.
9. Personal representational neglect – a relative impairment or inability to identify pictures of left hands compared to right hand.

Anosognosia [33–54]

1. Anosognosia for hemiparesis or hemiplegia – denial or gross underestimation of weakness or paralysis.
2. Anosodiaphoria – indifference or undue lack of concern for paretic arm or leg
3. Somatoparaphrenia – attribution of the left limb or limbs to another person.
4. Misoplegia – a hatred, extreme dislike and even acts of aggression toward the left limb or limbs.
5. Asomatognosia – denial of ownership of the left arm, less often the left.
6. Autotopagnosia – an inability to localize stimuli on a limb or different parts of the body.
7. Allesthesia – a mislocation of sensory stimuli within the same limb when stimulated.
8. Allochiria – a mislocation of the sensory stimulus to the opposite arm or leg.
9. Synchiria – a stimulus to one side of the body is perceived on both sides of the body.
10. Allokinesia – a request to move a limb is followed by moving the opposite limb to the one requested, representing the motor counterpart of the sensory syndrome of allochiria.
11. Supernumerary phantom limb – referred to as phantom third hand and an illusory sensation of the hand or arm in a position that is different to that of the actual paretic limb.
12. Xenomelia and apotemnophilia – expressed desire by the patient for amputation of healthy left arm or leg (occurs with a right superior parietal lesion).
13. Rubber hand illusion – when a person watches the stroking of an adjacent rubber hand at the same time that the person's own (hidden hand) is stroked this causes the relocation of the stroking sensation to the rubber hand.

Visuospatial Disorders

1. Visuomotor
2. Visuospatial

Aprosodia [55, 56]

1. Motor
2. Sensory
3. Global
4. Transcortical subtypes

Uncommon Right Hemisphere and Related Syndromes [57–78]

1. Apraxia of eye opening – eye closure with inability to open to command but may open spontaneously.
2. Response to next patient stimulation – patients responded to questions themselves when these were directed at patients near them or adjacent to them.
3. Topographical disorientation (TD) or geographical disorientation or planotopokinesia – sudden onset of losing one's bearings including for familiar places.
4. Empathy alteration (loss of empathy or hyper-empathy).
5. Gourmand syndrome – preoccupation with food and dining and has a correlation with impulse control disorders.
6. Hypergraphia, graphomimia, graphomania, and echographia – inappropriate and permanent writing behavior and a form of disinhibition syndrome secondary to release of left hemisphere writing activity.
7. Nosagnosia overestimation – exaggeration of the strength of unaffected limb may be present in association with right hemisphere syndromes, anosognosia, and hemineglect.
8. Musical ability alterations (discussed under newly acquired cultural circuits Chap. 12).

There exist other right hemisphere, frontal, and temporal network presentations that are not readily classifiable under the above system. Brain lesions may result in both hypo or hyperfunction of a circuit or cause hypo or hyperfunction remotely (diaschisis phenomenon). The theory of paradoxical functional facilitation proposes that one brain area reverses inhibition in other areas or in compensatory augmentation. This causes a counterintuitive paradoxical improvement in certain functions. Examples of such syndromes include the following:

- Emergent visual artistic ability in the setting of neurodegenerative disease especially with those affecting the left temporal lobe (progressive aphasia syndromes) such as has been reported in association with frontotemporal lobe disorders, stroke, Alzheimer's disease, Parkinson's, epilepsy, and migraine [79].
- Emergent literary artist ability especially with impairment of the right temporal lobe [80].
- Delusional misidentification syndromes, seen particularly with right frontal stroke [81].
- Increased humor, particularly after right frontal lesion such as stroke [82].

- Loss of visual imagery in dreaming [83].
- Savant syndromes that may include the sudden, acquired prodigious, sudden, splinter, or talented subtypes [84].

Delusional Misidentification Syndromes (DMIS) or Content-Specific Delusion Syndromes

These take the form whereby a person incorrectly identifies or duplicates persons, places, objects, or even events which may be learned by self-report or substantiated from family members or friends. Many different DMIS have been reported including the following:

1. *Capgras syndrome* – The belief by the person that a familiar individual or even the person themselves had been replaced by an imposter (hypoidentification).
2. *Fregoli's syndrome* – The belief that an individual familiar to the person is actually impersonating and is presenting themselves as a stranger (hyperidentification).
3. *Intermetamorphosis* – Two people, both familiar to the person, have interchanged identities with one another.
4. *Reduplicative paramnesias*

   (a) Place reduplication – The person is of the belief that there are two identical places sharing the same name but located in geographically distinct areas.
   (b) Chimeric – The person claims to be in their house when in fact they are lying in hospital, which may be considered to have been transformed into their own home.
   (c) Extravagant spatial localization – The person claims to be in a place different from the one at the time of interview, usually a place familiar to the person.

5. *De Clerambault's syndrome* – The belief that one is being loved by an individual belonging to higher socioeconomic status than self.
6. *Doppelgänger syndrome* – The belief that the person has a duplicate or twin.
7. *Othello syndrome* – The belief that the spouse is being unfaithful.
8. *Ekbom syndrome* (Parasitosis) – The belief of being infested or infected with insects.
9. *Cotard's syndrome* – The belief that one is actually demised.
10. *Dorian Gray syndrome* – The belief that one is immune to aging and is not actually aging.
11. *Lycanthropy* – The belief that there is a periodic transformation into an animal, most commonly a wolf.
12. *Incubus syndrome* – The belief that the person is visited by phantom lover.
13. *Picture syndrome* – The belief that persons in the news such as in newspapers or television are present in the home of the individual.
14. *Phantom boarder* – The belief that there is a guest in the person's home who is not welcomed there by the individual [85–97].

Most are diagnosed with Capgras or Fregoli' syndrome and not infrequently may be attributed to conditions such as schizophrenia, stroke, traumatic brain injury and dementia. The lesion in those presenting acutely is usually associated with a right frontal injury, but several reports of subcortical lesions, in particular the right caudate nucleus, have also been implicated [98].

References

1. Levy-Agresti J, Sperry RW. Differential perceptual capacities in major and minor hemispheries. Proc Natl Acad Sci U S A. 1968;61:1151.
2. Bear DM. Hemispheric specialization and the neurology of emotion. Arch Neurol. 1983;40:195–202.
3. Ross ED, Homan RW, Buck R. Differential hemispheric specialization of primary and social emotions. Neuropsychiatry Neurosurg Behav Neurol. 1994;7:1–19.
4. Joseph R. The right cerebral hemisphere: emotion, music, visuospatial skills, body image, dreams and awareness. J Clin Psychol. 1988;44:630–73.
5. Koch C. Consciousness. Cambridge, MA: MIT Press; 2012.
6. Mesulam M-M. Principles of behavioral and cognitive neurology. 2nd ed. Oxford: Oxford University Press; 2000.
7. Ely EW, Margolin R, Francis J, et al. Evaluation of delirium in critically ill patients: validation of the Confusion Assessment Method for the intenstive care unit (CAM-ICU). Crit Care Med. 2001;29(7):1370–9.
8. Kokmen E, Smith GE, Petersen RC, et al. The short test of mental status. Correlations with standardized psychometric testing. Arch Neurol. 1991;48:725–8.
9. Osterrieth PA. Le test de copie d'une figure complexe. Arch Psychol. 1944;30:206–356; Rey A. L'examen psychologique dans les cas d'encephalopathie traumatique. Archives de Psychologie 1941;28:286–340.
10. Possin KL, Laluz VR, Alcantar OZ, et al. Distinct neuroanatomical substrates and cognitive mechanisms of figure copy performance in Alzheimer's disease and behavioral variant fronto-temporal dementia. Neuropsychologia. 2011;49:43–8.
11. Strauss E, Spreen O. A comparison of the Rey and Taylor figures. Arch Clin Neuropsychol. 1990;5:417–20.
12. Randolph C. Manual: repeatable battery for the assessment of neuropsychological status. San Antonio: Psychological Corporation; 1998.
13. Cutting J. Study of anosognosia. J Neurol Neurosurg Psychiatry. 1978;41:548–55.
14. Pedersen PM, Henrik MA, Jorgensen HS, Nakayama H, Raaschou HO, Olsen TS. Frequency, determinants and consequences of anosognosia in acute stroke. J Neuroeng Rehabil. 1996;10:243–50.
15. Jehkonen M, Ahonen JP, Dastidar P, Koivisto AM, Laippala P, Vilkk J, Molnar G. Predictors of discharge to home during the first year after right hemisphere stroke. Acta Neurol Scand. 2001;104:136–4.
16. Maeshima S, Dohi N, Funahashi K, Mnakai K, Itakura T, Komai N. Rehabilitation of patients with anosognosia for hemiplegia due to intracerebral haemorrhage. Brain Inj. 1997;11:691–7.
17. Sacks O. The man who mistook his wife for a hat. Br J Psychiatry. 1995;166(1):130–1.
18. Bisiach E, Vallar G, Perani D, Papagno C, Berti A. Unawareness of disease following lesions of the right hemisphere: Anosognosia for hemiplegia and anosgnosia for hemianopia. Neuropsychologica. 1986;24:471–82.
19. Starkstein SE, Fedoroff JP, Price TR, Leiguarda R, Robinson RG. Anosognosia in patients with cerebrovascular lesions. A study of causative factors. Stroke. 1992;23:1446–53.
20. Cutting J. Study of anosognosia. J Neurol Neurourg Psychiatry. 1978;41:548–55.

21. Cocchini G, Beschin N, Fotopoulou A, Della SS. Explicit and implicit anosognosia or upper limb motor impairment. Neuropsychologia. 2010;48(5):1489–94.
22. Bergego C, Azouvi P, Samuel C, et al. Validation d'une e'chelle d'e'valuation fonction-nelle de l'he'mine'gligence dans la vie quotidienne: l'e'chelle CB. Ann Readapt Med Phys. 1995;38:183–9.
23. Hughlings JJ. On affections of speech from diseases of the brain. Brain. 1915;38:106–74.
24. Heilman KM, Scholes R, Watson RT. Auditory affective agnosia: disturbed comprehension of affective speech. J Neurol Neurosurg Psychiatry. 1975;38:69–72.
25. Edmondson JA, Ross ED, Chan JL, Seibert GB. The effect of right brain damage on acoustical measures of affective prosody in Taiwanese patients. J Phon. 1987;15:219–33.
26. Ross ED. Hemispheric specializations for emotions, affective aspects of language and communication and the cognitive control of display behaviors in humans. Prog Brain Res. 1996;107:583–94.
27. Shelton PA, Bowers D, Heilman KM. Peripersonal and vertical neglect. Brain. 1990;113:191–205.
28. Rapcsak SZ, Cimino CR, Heilman KM. Altitudinal neglect. Neurology. 1988;38(2):277–81.
29. Mark VW, Heilman KM. Diagonal spatial neglect. J Neurol Neurosurg Psychiatry. 1998;65(3):348–52.
30. Vuilleumier P, Valenza N, Mayer E, Reverdin A, Landis T. Near and far visual space in unilateral neglect. Ann Neurol. 1998;43(3):406–10.
31. Halligan PW, Marshall JC. Left neglect for near but not far space in man. Nature. 1991;350(6318):498–500.
32. Rapcsak SZ, Verfaellie M, Fleet WS, Heilman KM. Selective attention in hemispatial neglect. Arch Neurol. 1989;46(2):178–82.
33. Orfei MD, Robinson RG, Prigatano GP, et al. Anosognosia for hemiplegia after stroke is a multifaceted phenomenon: a systematic review of the literature. Brain. 2007;130:3075–90.
34. Garcin R, Varay A, Dimo H. Documentporu servier a l'etude des troubles du schema corporea. Rev Neurol. 1938;69:498–510.
35. Fotopoulou A, Rudd A, Holmes P, Kopelman M. Self observation reinstates motor awareness in anosognosia after hemiplegia. Neuropsychologia. 2009;47:1256–60.
36. Kortte KB, Hillis AE. Recent trends in rehabilitation interventions for visual neglect and anosognosia for hemiplegia following right hemisphere stroke. Future Neurol. 2011;6:33–43.
37. Appelros P, Karlsson GM, Seiger A, Nydevik I. Neglect and anosognosia after first-ever stroke: incidence and relationship to disability. J Rehabil Med. 2002;34:215–22.
38. Critchley M. The parietal lobes. London: Hafner Press; 1953.
39. Paulig M, Weber M, Garbelotto S. Somatoparaphrenia. A positive variant of anosognosia for hemiplegia. Nervenarzt. 2000;71(2):123–9.
40. Loetscher T, Regard M, Brugger P. Misoplegia: a review of the literature and a case without hemiplegia. J Neurol Neurosurg Psychiatry. 2006;77:1099–100.
41. Critchley M. Personification of paralysed limbs in hemiplegics. BMJ. 1955;2(4934):284–6; Critchley M. Misoplegia, or hatred of hemiplegia. Mt Sinai J Med. 1974;41:82–7
42. Feinberg T, Venneri A, Simone AM, et al. The neuroanatomy of asomatognosia and somatoparaphrenia. J Neurol Neurosurg Psychiatry. 2010;81:276–81.
43. Buxbaum LJ, Coslett HB. Specialised structural descriptions for human body parts: evidence from autotopagnosia. Cogn Neuropsychol. 2001;18:289–306.
44. Lepore M, Conson M, Grossi D, Trojano L. On the different mechanisms of spatial transpositions: a case of representational allochiria in clock drawing. Neuropsychologia. 2003;4:1290–5.
45. Venneri A, Pentore R, Cobelli M, Nichelli P, Shanks MF. Translocation of the embodied self without visuospatial neglect. Neuropsychologia. 2012;50(5):973–8.
46. Halligan PW, Marshall J, Wade D. Left on the right: allochiria in a case of left visuo-spatial neglect. J Neurol Neurosurg Psychiatry. 1992;55:717–9.
47. Young RR, Benson DF. Where is the lesion in allochiria. Arch Neurol. 1992;49:348–9.

48. Meador KJ, Allen ME, Adams RJ, Loring DW. Allochiria vs allesthesia. Is there a misperception? Arch Neurol. 1991;48(5):546–9.
49. Heilman KM, Valenstein E, Day A, Watson R. Frontal lobe neglect in monkeys. Neurology. 1995;45(6):1205–10.
50. Ehrenwald H. Anosgnosie und Depersonalisation. Nervenartzt. 1930;4:681–8.
51. McGeoch PD, Brang D, Song T, Lee RR, Huang M, Ramachandran VS. Xenomelia: a new right parietal lobe syndrome. J Neurol Neurosurg Psychiatry. 2011;82:1314–9.
52. Pasqualotto A, Proulx MJ. Two-dimensional rubber-hand illusion: the Dorian gray hand illusion. Multisens Res. 2015;28(1–2):101–10.
53. Ehrsson HH, Spence C, Passingham RE. That's my hand! Activity in premotor cortex reflects feeling of ownership of a limb. Science. 2004;305(5685):875–7.
54. Botvinick M, Cohen J. Rubber hands 'feel' touch that eyes see. Nature. 1998;391:756.
55. Gorelick PB, Ross ED. The aprosodias: further functional-anatomic evidence for the organization of affective language in the right hemisphere. J Neurol Neurosurg Psychiatry. 1987;50:553–60.
56. Ross ED. Modulation of affect and nonverbal communication by the right hemisphere. In: Principles of behavioural neurology. Philadelphia: Mesulam MM. FA Davis and Company; 1985.
57. Johnston JC, Rosenbaum DM, Picone CM, Grotta JC. Apraxia of eyelid opening secondary to right hemisphere infarction. Ann Neurol. 1989;25(6):622–4.
58. Lin Y-H, Liou L-M, Lai C-L, Chang Y-P. Right putamen hemorrhage manifesting as apraxia of eyelid opening. Neuropsychiatr Dis Treat. 2013;9:1495–7.
59. De Renzi E, Gentilini M, Bazolli C. Eyelid movement disorders and motor impersistence in acute hemisphere disease. Neurology. 1986;36(3):414–8.
60. Bogousslavsky J, Regli F. Response-to-next-patient-stimulation: a right hemisphere syndrome. Neurology. 1988;38(8):1225–7.
61. Barrash J. A historical review of topographical disorientation and its neuroanatomical correlates. J Clin Exp Neuropsychol. 1998;20(6):807–27.
62. Hirayama K, Taguchi Y, Sato M, Tsukamoto T. Limbic encephalitis presenting with topographical disorientation and amnesia. J Neurol Neurosurg Psychiatry. 2003;74(1):110–2.
63. Richard-Mornas A, Mazzietti A, Koenig O, et al. Emergence of hyper empathy after right amygdalohippocampectomy. Neurocase. 2013; https://doi.org/10.1080/1355479 4.2013.826695.
64. Regard M, Landis T. "Gourmand syndrome": eating passion associated with right anterior lesions. Neurology. 1998;50(3):831.
65. Yamadori A, Mori E, Tabuchi M, Kudo Y, Mitani Y. Hypergraphia: a right hemisphere syndrome. J Neurol Neurosurg Psychiatry. 1986;49(10):1160–4.
66. Carota A, Annoni JM, Combremont P, Clarke S, Bogousslavsky J. Hypergraphia, verbal aspontaneity and post-stroke depression secondary to right cingulate and corpus callosum infarction. J Neurol. 2003;250(4):508–10.
67. Panico A, Parmegriani A, Trimble MR. Compulsive painting: a variant of hypergraphia? Neurology. 1996;9(3):177–80.
68. Gil R, Neau JP, Aubert I, Fabre C, Agbo C, Tantot AM. Anosognosic graphomimia: an uncommon variety of hypergraphia in right sylvian infarction. Rev Neurol (Paris). 1995;151(3):198–201.
69. Cambier J, Masson C, Benammou S, Robine B. Graphomania. Compulsive graphic activity as a manifestation of fronto-callosal glioma. Rev Neurol (Paris). 1988;144(3):158–64.
70. Nimmo-Smith I, Marcel AJ, Tegnér R. A diagnostic test of unawareness of bilateral motor task abilities in anosognosia for hemiplegia. J Neurol Neurosurg Psychiatry. 2005;76(8):1167–9.
71. Andre JM, Beis JM, Morin N, Paysant J. Buccal hemineglect. Arch Neurol. 2000;57(12):1734–41.
72. Mallory PF, Richardson ED. Frontal lobes and content specific delusions. J Neuropsychiatr. 1994;6:455–66.

73. Feinberg TE. Delusional Misidentification. Psychiatr Clin N Am. 2005;28:665–6683.
74. Ramachandran VS. Consciousness and body image: lessons from phantom limbs, Capgras syndrome and pain asymbolia. Philos Times R Soc Lond B. 1998;353:1851–9.
75. Sinkman A. The syndrome of capgras. Psychiatry. 2008;71(4):371–7.
76. Collins MN. Capgras' syndrome with organic disorders. Postgrad Med J. 1990;66:1064–7.
77. Hakim H. Pathogenesis of reduplicative paramnesia. J Neurol Neurosurg Psychiatry. 1988;51:839–41.
78. Hirstein W. Capgras syndrome: a novel probe for understanding the neural representation of the identity and familiarity of persons. Proc R Soc Lond B. 1997;264:437–44.
79. Schott GD. Pictures as a neurological tool: lessons from enhanced and emergent artistry in brain disease. Brain. 2012;135:1947–63.
80. Miller B. The frontotemporal lobe dementias. New York: Oxford University Press; 2013.
81. Christodoulou GN, Magariti M, Kontaxakis VP, Christodoulou NG. The delusion misidentification syndromes: strange, fascinating and instructive. Curr Pyschiatry Rep. 2009;11:185–9.
82. Pell MD. Judging emotion and attitutdes from prosody following brain damage. Prog Brain Res. 2006;156:303–17.
83. Pen'a-Casanova J, Roig-Rovira T, Bermudez A, Tolosa-Sarro E. Optic aphasia, optic apraxia and loss of dreaming. Brain Lang. 1985;26:63–71.
84. Treffert DA. Islands of genius. London: Jessica Kingsley Publishers; 2010.
85. Mallory PF, Richardson ED. Frontal lobes and content specific delusions. J Neuropsychiatr. 1994;6:455–66.
86. Feinberg TE. Delusional misidentification. Psychiatr Clin N Am. 2005;28:665–6683.
87. Ramachandran VS. Consciousness and body image: lessons from phantom limbs, Capgras syndrome and pain asymbolia. Philos Times R Soc Lond B. 1998;353:1851–9.
88. Sinkman A. The syndrome of capgras. Psychiatry. 2008;71(4):371–7.
89. Collins MN. Capgras' syndrome with organic disorders. Postgrad Med J. 1990;66:1064–7.
90. Hakim H. Pathogenesis of reduplicative paramnesia. J Neurol Neurosurg Psychiatry. 1988;51:839–41.
91. Hirstein W. Capgras syndrome: a novel probe for understanding the neural representation of the identity and familiarity of persons. Proc R Soc Lond B. 1997;264:437–44.
92. Moriyama Y. Fregoli syndrome Accompanied with Prosopagnosia in a women with a 40-year History of Schizophrenia. Keio J Med. 2007;56(4):130–4.
93. Kapur N, Turner A, King C. Reduplicative Paramnesia: possible anatomical and neuropsychological mechanisms. J Neurol Neurosurg Psychiatry. 1988;51:579–81.
94. Feinberg TE, Roane DM. Misidentification syndromes. In: Feinberg TE, MJH F, editors. Behavioral neurology and neuropsychology. New York: McGraw Hill; 1997.
95. Aziz MA, Razik GN, Donn JE. Dangerousness and management of delusional misidentification syndrome. Psychopathology. 2005;38(2):97–102. Epub 2005
96. Devinsky O. Delusional misidentification s and duplications: right brain lesions, left brain delusions. Neurology. 2009;72:80–7.
97. Larner AJ. Delusion of pregnancy in frontotemporal lobar degeneration with motor neurone diseases. Behav Neurol. 2008;19:199–200.
98. Forstl H, Almeida OP, Owen AM, Burns A, Howard R. Psychiatric, neurological and medical aspects of misidentification syndromes: a review of 260 cases. Psychol Med. 1991;21(4):905–10.
99. Vincent JL, Kahn I, Snyder AC, et al. Evidence for a frontoparietal control system revealed by intrinsic functional connectivity. J Neurophysiol. 2008;100(6):3328–42.

Chapter 10
Left Dominant Perisylvian Network for Language Syndromes (and Language ICN Network)

From a philosophical point of view, it is difficult to separate thought and language. Although we may think silently, also termed inner speech (endophasia), we can both speak and write our thoughts, also termed exophasia. Gardiner appropriately termed thoughts and words as the "mental commerce of the mind" [1]. Another language researcher, Brain, considered language and words as "the guardians of our thoughts" [2]. Language and speech in that language, if impaired (dysphasia), are attributable to a left-brain lesion in most people, and speech impairment or dysarthria is consequent to an extracerebral derangement often due to cranial nerve impairment or speech musculature or due to vocal cord disturbance. In brief the neurobiology of language components and related activities can be summarized as follows:

- Thoughts – mental activity reflected in a linguistic or nonlinguistic form
- Endophasia – inner or internal language
- Exophasia – spoken or written language
- Ideas – encoding of thoughts into sounds or utterances with the ideas pertaining to events, objects, and actions and employing verbal symbols for transmission to another person
- Language – communicable part of a person's knowledge and a signaling system used by one person to communicate with others
- Speech – oral communication subserved by coordinated muscular activity with the neural controlling networks
- Grammar – rules that determine vocal sounds and combine to form words (lexicon), phrases, sentences. Grammar may be divided into the following:

  - Phonology – phonemes or sounds
  - Morphology – morphemes or words
  - Grapheme – the smallest meaningful unit in writing
  - Semantics – the symbolic meaning associated with a word or phrase
  - Syntax – sentence construction

© Springer Nature Switzerland AG 2020
M. Hoffmann, *Clinical Mentation Evaluation*,
https://doi.org/10.1007/978-3-030-46324-3_10

A The language-relevant connectome

- Arcuate fasc. (long)
- Arcuate fasc. (ant)
- Arcuate fasc. (post)
- Inf. frontal-occipital fasc.
- frontal aslant tract
- inf. logitudinal fasc.
- uncinate fasc.

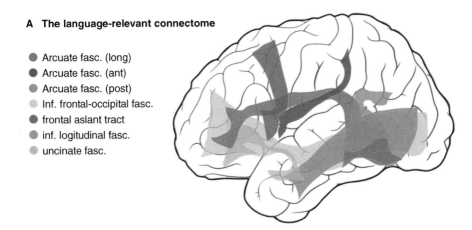

Fig. 10.1 Language connectome. (Figure with permission Hagoort [15])

Functional imaging (fMRI, PET, magnetoencephalography) of language-related activity has revealed extensive participatory circuits including subcortical components, the basal nuclei, thalamus, and the anterior and inferior temporal lobes (Fig. 10.1), as well as activation of both hemispheres, albeit left more than the right. Perhaps, because of the extensive circuitry involved, MR- and CT-based perfusion scanning have revealed that this modality is a better predictor of the aphasic-type syndrome and extent of deficit compared to Diffusion weighted imaging (DWI) [3].

The extensive language connectome reveals widespread activation by functional imaging well beyond the perisylvian language network with the familiar Broca's and Wernicke's areas. In summary these areas include the following:

- Auditory: bilateral superior temporal lobe gyrus and Heschl's gyrus
- Visual: left inferior occipital lobe gyrus
- Phonologic networks: left superior temporal lobe gyrus, supramarginal gyrus
- Semantic evaluation: left middle temporal lobe gyrus, angular gyrus
- Short-term memory (auditory, verbal): left supramarginal gyrus and superior temporal gyrus
- Word retrieval: left frontal opercular, middle and inferior temporal gyrus, angular gyrus
- Phonologic output: left superior temporal lobe gyrus and supramarginal gyrus
- Speech production: Broca's area, putamen located bilaterally, and motor cranial nerve nuclei
- Written language: superior parietal region, left angular gyrus, middle frontal (Exner's area)
- Sentence assembly: left frontal operculum
- Syntax assembly: left dorsolateral prefrontal cortex
- Conceptual and semantic components integration: bilateral anterior temporal lobes [4]

Language Dominance and Accompanying Domains Such as Apraxias

Left handedness occurs in approximately 10% of the population and is associated with left hemisphere dominance in ~70% with only 30% having right brain dominance for language. Left-handed people are more likely to develop aphasia with stroke, implying greater propensity for bilateral language representation. The aphasia tends to be milder and recovery of aphasia is more rapid [5]. Additional language acquisitions also influence the recovery trajectory. Aphasia in polyglots after stroke often follows the rules of Ribot and Pitres.

- *Ribot's law*: better performance in the native language as opposed to the newly acquired language
- *Pitres law*: the more frequently used language prior to stroke onset often recovers better.

Crossed aphasia occurs rarely (~1% of the time) and may be seen in right-handed people who develop aphasia after injury to the right hemisphere rather than the usual left hemisphere-associated aphasic syndromes [6] (Fig. 10.2).

The Clinical Aphasia Syndromes May Be Conveniently Parcellated into Four Principal Functions Yielding a Clinical Classification System of Eight Different Types (Fig. 10.3)

These include fluency, comprehension, repetition, and naming deficits. The mildest forms of aphasia present only with dysnomia. This remains an overly simplistic approach as patients with expressive, Broca's aphasia generally also have some degree of comprehension deficits and as with Wernicke's aphasia where some degree of expressive difficulty may also be present.

Clinical Aphasia Subtypes Classification

Perisylvian Aphasias

- Broca's
- Wernicke's
- Conduction

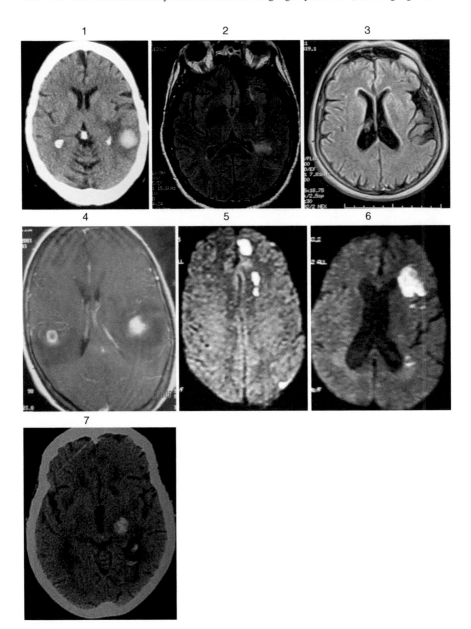

Fig. 10.2 Different aphasia presentations. Wernicke's – 1, conduction – 2, primary progressive aphasia – 3, pure word deafness – 4, aphemia – 5, transcortical motor aphasia – 6, subcortical aphasia – 7

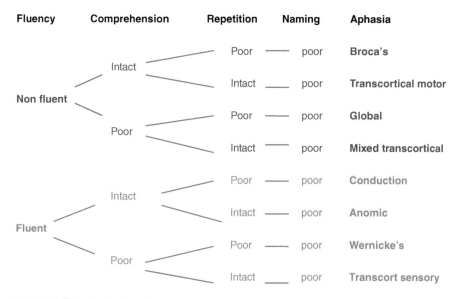

Fig. 10.3 Clinical aphasia subtypes

Extra Perisylvian

- Transcortical motor
- Transcortical sensory
- Transcortical mixed

Very Large and Very Small Lesions Causing Aphasia

- Global aphasia
- Anomic aphasia

Subcortical Aphasias

- Thalamic
- White matter
- Internal capsule
- Caudate

Anomias are by definition mild aphasic syndromes with preserved comprehension, fluency, and repetition, but confrontation naming and word generation tests may be impaired (Fig. 10.4).

Fig. 10.4 Broca's (blue), conduction (red), and Wernicke's (green) aphasia approximate lesion sites

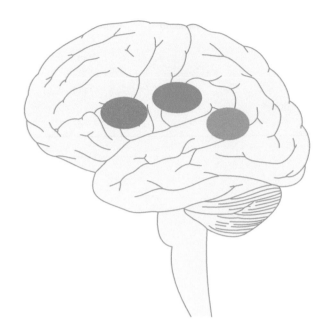

Anomias are the most commonly encountered language deficits and are part of all aphasic syndromes. Dysnomia affects mostly nouns, but can also affect verbs and adjectives. Dysnomia occurs with many neurological illness (stroke, toxic and infectious encephalopathies, dementia, delirium) and even overlaps with normality (tip of the tongue phenomenon). Dysnomias are considered to be a very sensitive test for overall neurological cognitive status but are not specific with respect to cause. A simplified anomia classification with approximate anatomic hubs is depicted in Fig. 10.5.

- Word production anomia – inability to name but with cueing is able to name correctly
- Word selection anomia – inability to name and even with cueing is unable to name correctly but still can select correct object from a group
- Semantic anomia – a combination of the first two anomias with inability to name, unable to benefit from cueing, and is not able to single out the object when given the correct name [7, 8]

Other less common syndromes and those related to aphasias may include the following.

Fig. 10.5 Transcortical motor (pink), transcortical sensory (orange), and transcortical mixed (purple) aphasia approximate lesion sites

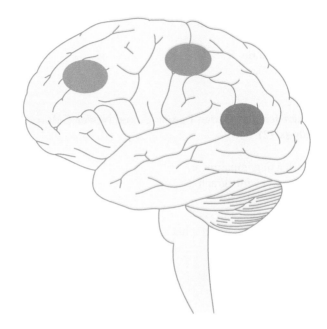

Other Aphasias and Related Syndromes

- Mutism
- Aphemia – muteness but able to write
- Foreign accent syndrome – acquired accent change due to motor aphasia or cranial nerve damage
- Forced hyperphasia – urge to read all signs and verbiage in the immediate environment
- Dynamic aphasia of Luria
- Pure word-deafness and auditory agnosia – can hear environmental sounds but not speech
- Gerstmann's syndrome – acalculia, right left disorientation, finger anomia, agraphia
- Angular gyrus syndrome – same as Gerstmann's but with addition of dysnomia and alexia
- Ictal aphasia – seizure-related language impairment
- Acquired stuttering
- Echolalia and palilalia

Allied Speech Disorders

- Dysarthria
- Aphonia

Disorders of Written Language and Newer Cultural Abilities (see Chap. 12)

- Reading impairment
- Alexia with agraphia
- Central alexia
- Semantic paralexia
- Alexia without agraphia
- Agraphia
- Acalculia

Bedside Testing for Aphasia Syndromes

Bedside testing (Language version of the Coconuts Test, Chapter (5)) [9]

Speech and Language Assessment

Scoring: 1 for each error, 0 is normal. Any point lost in any of the 8 items constitutes anabnormality for that category

Speech and language – score 1 for each error, 0 is normal

Naming: Name 3 objects (pen, watch, ID card) and name 3 colors /6

Fluency: grade as fluent (0), non-fluent (1), mute (2) /2

Comprehension: Close your eyes, squeeze my hand. Score 1 for each failure /2

Repetition: "Today is a sunny and windy day." No word repeated (2), partial (1), all (0) /2

Write a sentence. What is your job? Must contain subject and verb and makes sense /3

Reading: "Close your eyes." No words read (2), partial (1), or all words (0) /2

Motor Speech

Dysarthria. During interview, are words slurred? Nil (0), mild slurring (1), marked slurring (2)/2

Hypophonia: normal (0), voice softer than normal (1), very low volume, barely audible (2) /2

Total Score /21

Fig. 10.6 Word
production (dark blue),
word selection (pink),
and semantic anomia
(light blue) approximate
lesions sites

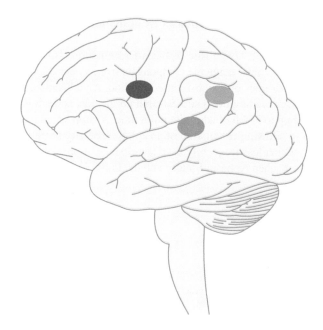

Metric Testing

Boston Naming Test (BNT) Version 2

This is a very popular and widely used language test that may be viewed as a language metric screening test. This booklet form consists of 60 simple line drawings graded into 20 easy, 20 moderately difficult, and 20 more difficult items. Two versions are present in the booklet: a full-length 60-item test and a short 15-item one (Fig. 10.6). Both have a cueing option consisting of 4 semantic cueing items presented on the back of each line drawing, with gender-, education-, and age-specific norms available. A typical normal adult score for the 60-item test is 52 +/−3 [10].

The Western Aphasia Battery (WAB-Revised)

The focus of this test is in arriving at a clinical aphasia classification through metric assessments. The domains include expressive, receptive, global transcortical (motor sensory, mixed), and anomic aphasia subtypes. An overall score, termed aphasia quotient (100 is the maximum score) and cortical quotient, is calculated to assist with monitoring progress or deterioration over time which is very helpful in guiding the rehabilitative process [11].

Boston Diagnostic Aphasia Examination (Version 3)

The Boston Diagnostic Aphasia Examination (BADE version 3) focuses more on the individual language components from a neurobiological perspective rather than a syndrome- or lesion-focused method. An advantage is that it is a comprehensive test, consisting of 34 subtests, but on the downside, it is a time demanding test, taking up to 3–4 h of administration time. A short version can be completed within 1 h, also allowing calculation of an aphasia severity score [12].

Other less frequently used tests that are more popular in aphasia research include the Aachen Aphasia Battery and the Porch Index of Communicative Ability (PICA) [13, 14].

References

1. Gardiner AH. The theory of speech and language. Westport CT: Greenwood Press; 1979.
2. Brain R. Speech disorders. Aphasia, apraxia and agnosia. Butterworth: Oxford; 1967.
3. Hillis AE, Barker PB, Beauchamp NJ, Gordon B, Wityk RJ. MR perfusion imaging reveals regions of hypoperfusion associated with aphasia and neglect. Neurology. 2000;55(6):782–8.
4. Hillis AE. Aphasia. Progress in the last quarter of a century. Neurology. 2007;69:200–13.
5. Wuillemin D, Richardson B, Lynch J. Right hemisphere involvement in processing later learned languages in multilinguals. Brain Lang. 1994;46:620–36.
6. Mariën P, Paghera B, De Deyn PP, Vignolo LA. Adult crossed aphasia in dextrals revisited. Review Cortex. 2004;40(1):41–74.
7. Geschwind N. The varieties of naming errors. Cortex. 1967;3:97–112.
8. Goodglass H, Wingfield A. Word finding deficits in aphasia: brain-behavior relations and clinical symptomatology. In: Goodglass H, Wingfield A, editors. Anomia: Neuroanatomical and cognitive correlates. San Diego: Academic Press; 1997.
9. Hoffmann M, Schmitt F, Bromley E. Comprehensive cognitive neurological assessment in stroke. Acta Neurol Scand. 2009;119:162–71.
10. Kaplan EF, Goodglass H, Weintraub S. The Boston naming test. 2nd ed. Philadelphia: Lea and Febiger; 1983.
11. Kertesz A. Western aphasia battery revised. Examiner's manual. Pearson: San Antonio; 2007.
12. Goodglass H, Kaplan E, Barresi B. The Boston diagnostic aphasia examination (BDAE-3). 3rd ed. Pearson: San Antonio; 2000.
13. Huber W, Weniger D, Poeck K, Willmes K. The Aachen aphasia test rationale and construct validity. Nervenarzt. 1980;51(8):475–8.
14. Phillips PP, Halpin G. Language impairment evaluation in aphasic patients: developing more efficient measures. Arch Phys Med Rehabil. 1978;59(7):327–30.
15. Hagoort P. The neurobiology of language beyond single word processing. Science. 2019;366:55–8.

Chapter 11
Occipitotemporal Network for Face and Object Recognition Syndromes (Visual Network) Occipitoparietal and Provincial Hub Syndromes

Approximately half of the human cerebral cortex is concerned with vision, and it usually supersedes other senses when there is conflict with other sensory inputs. Our visual system has developed predominance over the other senses, and vision focuses our attention. It has been hypothesized that attention is nature's way of coping with the prodigious sensory input receiving a constant stream of information. We are subject to a profusion of sensory input, with the combined human sensory inputs receiving ~11 million bits of information per second. However, we can only process ~16–50 bits per second (0.0002%). The majority of decisions are therefore made at a non-conscious level [1, 2].

The cerebral vision areas, V1 (BA 17), V2 (BA 18), and V3 (BA 19), subserve binocular vision, line orientation, contrast, and brightness. Areas further along the ventral and dorsal visual streams process information from progressively more basic features, such as overall shape and form, to intermediate functions, such as depth perception, and finally to higher-level vision, such as object and face interpretation. Area V4 is concerned with color vision (V4v, ventral component) and size evaluation (V4d, dorsal component) and V5 motion processing. Area V6 subserves three-dimensional vision, self-motion analysis, visual guidance during reaching, and finger pointing. Area V7, which lies within the posterior intraparietal sulcus, has foveal representations and is involved in saccadic eye and reaching movements. V8 is associated with color interpretation separate from V4 [3–7] (Fig. 11.1). Cytoarchitectonic studies and functional imaging by MRI scanning has revealed over 30 different visual areas within the human brain [8]. These may be variously impacted by the lesions affecting the visual networks. Stroke is a common cause of visual disturbance but other processes such as eclampsia, posterior reversible encephalopathy syndrome (PRES), and leukoaraiosis may also often present with vision disorders (Fig. 11.2). In view of the extensive human visual network, a convenient manner of reviewing the manifold presentations is according to the principal visual networks of the brain ((Fig. 11.3) and (Table 11.1)). Remarkable congruence of these clinically known and cytoarchitectonic networks has also been recorded by recent functional MRI intrinsic connectivity scans (ICN) (Fig. 11.4).

© Springer Nature Switzerland AG 2020
M. Hoffmann, *Clinical Mentation Evaluation*,
https://doi.org/10.1007/978-3-030-46324-3_11

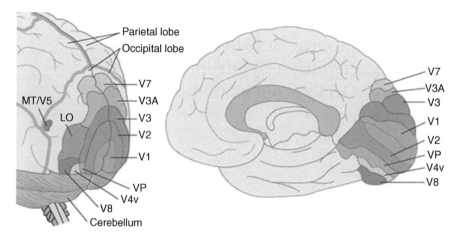

Fig. 11.1 Visual cortical areas. (Figure with permission Barrett et al. [47])

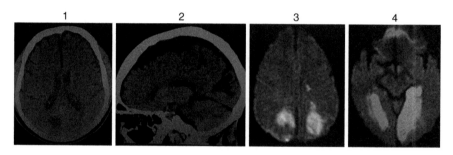

Fig. 11.2 Right mesial occipital infarct (1, 2), bilateral parieto-occipital lesions due to posterior reversible encephalopathy syndrome (PRES) presenting with simultanagnosia (3) and bioccipital infarcts, cortical blindness, and Anton's syndrome (4)

A Classification of the Principal Circuits Relating to Visual Disorders and Topological and Hodological Circuitry Phenomena (Fig. 11.3)

1. Elementary cortical areas, BA 17–19 (V1, V2, V3)
2. Ventral stream (what) related syndromes
3. Dorsal stream (where) related syndromes
4. Occipitoparietal (when) stream related syndromes
5. Occipitotemporal amygdala and related syndromes
6. Occipitoinferior frontal and related syndromes

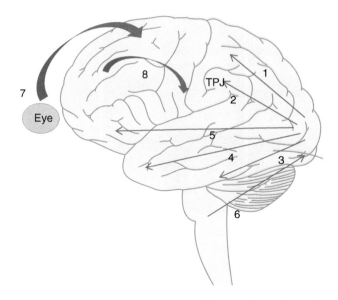

Fig. 11.3 Visual radiations: 1. dorsal occipitoparietal (where), 2. occipitoparietal (when), 3. occipitotemporal (what), 4. occipitotemporal amygdala, 5. occipitofrontal (via extreme and external capsule), 6. brainstem (peduncular hallucinations) (remote), and 7. ocular (Charles Bonnet syndrome). 8. Top-down influence on perception

Table 11.1 Visual disorders and syndromes associated with more elementary cortical areas, BA 17–19 (V1, V2, V3)

1. Hemianopias, scotomas – Visual field deficits and central vision deficits
2. Simple hallucinations – See simple shapes, colors, phosphenes (light or colors in absence of light stimulation), photopsia (lights, sparks on colors due to mechanical or electrical stimulation), teichopsia (patterns or zig zag lines) or visual snow
3. Complex hallucinations – Seeing people or landscapes
4. Visual apperceptive agnosia (visual form agnosia) – Unable to identify simple line drawings
5. Visual associative agnosia – Unable to identify objects visually but can by tactile and auditory
6. Perceptual categorization defect – Difficulty in recognizing objects seen in unusual angles [9]
7. Cortical blindness – Unable to see secondary to bilateral occipital lesions, usually infarcts
8. Anton's syndrome – Cortical blindness but denies the deficit [10]
9. Inverse Anton's syndrome – Denial of visual perception and maintain they are blind but require no assistance due to disconnection of parietal lobe attentional circuitry from visual perception
10. Blindsight – Cortical blindness but with intact discrimination ability
11. Riddoch' syndrome – Akin to cortical blindness, with bilateral (or hemifield blindness), can only see people, for example when they move, the V5 motion cortex being intact [11, 12]. The moving objects have little detail such as color
12. Gnosanopsia – Awareness only of the movement without visual perception of it
13. Scieropia – Overall dimming, or general darkening of environment [13]
14. Astereopsis – Loss of depth perception

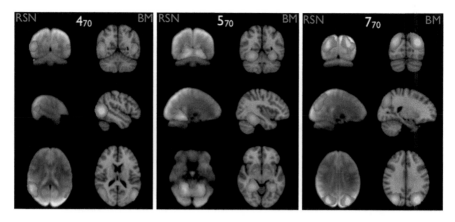

Fig. 11.4 Visual ICN network. Map 4_{70} corresponds to area V5 (motion), map 5_{70} covers the ventral/ventrolateral visual stream, and map 7_{70} covers the dorsal visual stream. (Figure with permission Smith et al. [48])

7. Lesions outside the cortex affecting vision – Charles Bonnet (retinal disease) and peduncular hallucinosis (brainstem lesion)
8. Prefrontal top-down attentional control of vision

Occipitoparietal (When) Pathway

Assessment of motion and estimation of objects in the environment are the functions of the "when" pathway (Table 11.2). This allows assessment of the overall temporal order of events as well as whether events have occurred simultaneously or not (Table 11.3). The right parietal lobe contains part of the visual occipitoparietal stream and is dominant for the overall temporal order of events and subserves both visual fields [22–24].

1. Chronoataraxis refers to the loss of sense of time and includes (i) inability to judge the passage of time (example length of interview), (ii) altered temporal relation of habitual activities (brushing teeth, showering), (iii) whether time appears to pass more quickly, and (iv) illusory acceleration of moving objects (quick motion or Zeitraffer phenomenon) [15].

Occipitotemporal Cortex and Pathway (Fig. 11.5)

Critical social information and information such as people's facial expression and their meaning are conveyed by this tract with includes the amygdala mediating fear and aggression, for example. Syndromes related to the occipitotemporal fiber tract include the following:

Table 11.2 Ventral stream disorders [14, 15]

1. Achromatopsia – Selective loss of color vision. Often report that everything looks like shades of gray
2. Color anomia – Fail to correctly name colors on visual presentation (not due to aphasia or color perception). It is a two-way deficit as one cannot name colors when presented colored stimuli nor point to the color when given their name
3. Color agnosia (agnosia is "non-knowledge," from Greek) – Unable to name or distinguish colors or name them but are able to read Ishihara plates as they have normal color perception
4. Hyperchromatopsia – increased activity in color cortex
5. Color hallucinations and illusions
6. Prosopagnosia – Able to discern all facial features but unable to recognize familiar faces
7. Facial hallucinations and illusions
8. Facial intermetamorphosia – a change in the visual perception of face identification
9. Prosopometamorphosia – Illusions of distorted faces
10. Visual object agnosia – Inability to identify the percept at all, for example that a bird is a bird
11. Object hallucinations and illusions – May involve reading and text hallucinations
12. Optic anomia or aphasia – Visual naming deficit with normal tactile and auditory naming ability
13. Environmental agnosia – Inability to recognize familiar places
14. Landscape hallucinations
15. Micropsia (size and object distortion or metamorphopsia) – Objects appear smaller
16. Macropsia (size and object distortion or metamorphopsia) – Objects appear larger
17. Pelopsia – Objects appear closer
18. Telopsia – Objects appear further away
19. Synesthesia – Merging of sensory inputs (colored hearing, colored music, colored grapheme)
20. Pareidolia – Illusory images of faces or specific objects seen as visual patterns when viewing clouds or plants for example, thought to be due to a hyperconnection of visual areas [16]
21. Lilliputian hallucinations – Seeing people, birds, carriages, and buildings in smaller size

1. *Post-traumatic stress disorder (PTSD)*: This syndrome includes reliving previously stressful events, associated with flashbacks often with strong emotional experiences, vivid memory incursions, recurring dreams, visual hallucinations, hyperarousal and associated autonomic activity. This occipito-amydaloid hyperconnectivity syndrome represents an example of hodological hyperconnection [25, 26].

2. *Klüver-Bucy syndrome*: This complex temporal lobe syndrome has prominent components of visual agnosia in people not recognizing objects and expressing no fear of snakes, for example (primates). In addition, there is a placidity, at times hypersexuality and a hyperorality, with placing of objects in their mouth. The critical lesions include anterior temporal lobe lesions, or lesions along the occipitotemporal tracts.

3. *Kalopsia and kakopsia*: These Greek-derived words (kalos – seeing items as beautiful or comforting and opsis and kakos – unpleasant or bad) refer to pleasant and unpleasant subjective experiences, respectively, in response to certain visual perceptions. These may be explained by a hodological hyperfunction between the emotional brain networks, especially the amgydala and the visual cortex [15, 27].

Table 11.3 Dorsal stream syndromes [14, 15, 17, 18]

1. Dorsal and ventral simultanagnosia – Fragmentation of visual field or piecemeal vision
2. Optic ataxia – Impaired target pointing using visual guidance
3. Oculomotor apraxia – Impairment of directing gaze at a new stimulus (a visual scanning deficit)
4. Balint's syndrome – The combination of simultanagnosia, optic ataxia, and optic apraxia
5. Polyopia – Multiple images of a single object are seen
6. Entomopia – Variant of polyopia, seeing multiple copies of a grid-like pattern
7. Akinetopsia – Selective loss of motion vision
8. Cinematographic vision – Perceived visual discontinuity of movement with the impression of a series of still images seen with some dysfunctional movie films
9. Palinopsias – Persistence of the visual appreciation of the image of an object after it has disappeared
10. Delayed palinopsia – Image of the object returns or its recurrence when it is no longer present
11. Illusory visual spread – The design or motif of object spreads to the adjacent areas
12. Trailing phenomenon – The experience of stationary items, images, or objects trailing a moving item, a type of visual perseveration
13. Negative hallucination
14. Visual allesthesia – The visual field is tilted, inverted, or rotated
15. Inverted vision – Upside-down vision, as it may occur with Wallenberg brainstem stroke syndrome
16. Autoscopy – Out of body experience with the projection of one's body or face above or from an external point of view typically lasting from seconds to minutes
17. Heautoscopy – Out of body experience whereby one sees oneself
18. Extracampine hallucinations
19. Oculogyric illusion – A visual vestibular disorders of paroxysmal perceptual alterations
20. Oculogravic – A visual vestibular disorders with ostensible movement of one's visual field during acceleration due to gravity, for example experienced by pilots
21. Zingerle's automatosis – Visual hallucination in association with vestibular impairment [19]
22. Paroxysmal perceptual alteration (PPA) – Text or other visual pattern is briefly intensified [20, 21]

Fig. 11.5
Occipitotemporal pathway.
(Figure with permission
Catani et al. [49])

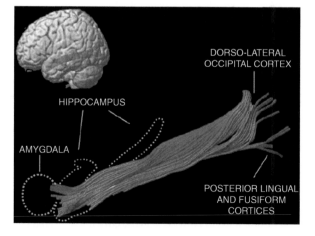

Occipitofrontal Fasciculus Via the Extreme and External Capsule (Fig. 11.6)

1. Content-specific delusions (delusional misidentification syndromes) – refers to a range of differing delusions mostly associated with right frontal lesions. Some occur more commonly, such as the Capgras syndrome (delusion that someone close to them has been replaced by an imposter) and Fregoli syndrome (a person familiar to the person takes on the appearance of a stranger). With the network for facial recognition remaining intact, the circuitry mediating the emotional responses and associations is impaired. It is a perceptual processing abnormality rather than a disorder of thinking. Viewed in this way, the Capgras syndrome may be regarded as opposite to prosopagnosia. The processing tracts for face recognition remains intact, but the tracts that mediate the emotional responses to the particular face are not functional [28].

2. Anoneria – Cerebral lesions (strokes, tumors, infections) may at times target the neural circuitry that mediates dreaming. The visual imagery or visual memory–related syndromes such as anoreria and Charcot–Wilbrand syndromes may be explained by the topographical or hodological pathophysiological features of the lesion. The clinical syndrome of Charcot's variant is characterized by dreams of specific faces, movement, or colors. Wilbrand's variant or global anoreria is a syndrome whereby there is complete absence of dreaming. Anoneirognosis is a syndrome where there is a reality-dream/reality confusional state. Described causes have included carbon monoxide poisoning, dementias, stroke, and cerebral trauma with mostly bilateral occipitotemporal lesions [29, 30].

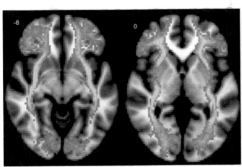 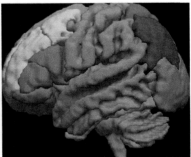

The inferior fronto-occipital fasciculus (IFOF) is the longest associative bundle in the human brain and connects parts of the occipital cortex, temporo-basal, superior parietal lobule to the frontal lobe. It traverses through the external/extreme capsule complex

Cortical regions connected by the IFOF (Montreal Neurological Institute Map). Light green: superior frontal, yellow: rostral and caudal frontal cortex; red: pars operularis, triangularis and orbitofrontal PFC, dark blue: lateral, medial portions of OFPFC, pink: superior parietal gyrus; green: angular gyrus; orange: occipital lobe; teal: fusiform gyrus.

Fig. 11.6 Inferior fronto-occipital fasciculus (IFOF). (Figure credit Caverzasi et al. [50])

Remote Effects: Tract 7 (Fig. 11.3)

1. *Charles Bonnet syndrome (CBS)*: This reports of complex visual hallucinations in the context of anterior or ocular vision impairment or blindness. This syndrome may represent a type of denervation hypersensitivity or hodological-type hyperactivation. The visual hallucinations are usually Lilliputian type (diminutive in appearance) of people, or objects, lasting 3–5 min, several times per day. Insight that these hallucinations are not real is preserved and they are confined to the visual domain [31].
2. *Peduncular hallucinations*: These are visual hallucinations that appear after a brainstem lesion, typically infarcts. They are realistic to the person, usually occur during night time, and are vivid and colorful. The mechanism is presumed similar to the hallucinations that may occur during normal REM sleep and related to the ascending reticular activating system [32].

Top-Down Influences – Prefrontal

The prefrontal cortex (PFC) is the primary initiator of top-down attentional control required in object perception. The PFC is implicated in continuing goal-related information and in delegating attentional resources for both selection and set shifting. Attention is a key neurophysiological requirement for visual processing, having both voluntary and involuntary components.

1. *Change blindness*: For example, changes in the successive presentation of a photograph or picture frequently go unnoticed by the viewer, which is attributed to the fragmented nature of our attentional abilities [33].
2. *Inattention blindness*: This involves a failure to recognize an object or event that may be in plain sight, which is attributed to our attentional systems being required to focus elsewhere [27]. This has been particularly well illustrated by the Invisible "Gorilla Test" of Chabris and Simon (http://www.theinvisiblegorilla.com/gorilla_experiment.html) [34, 35].
3. *Perceptual change without any sensory stimulation*: With bistable figures such as the Rubin vase, the alternating perception of such figures, oscillating between two faces or a vase, may not occur with various prefrontal lesions [36, 37].

Clinical Bedside and Metric Testing

When reported symptoms trigger a visual related symptom, direct questioning and inquiry as to the large number of visual hallucinations is required. Most of these will rely on history, for example the various illusions and subjective phenomena.

Evaluation of basic visual processing is required before progressing to more complex visual disorders evaluation. Assessment of visual acuity by Snellen charts or similar tests as well as visual field assessment by 4 quadrant confrontation testing or computerized perimetry, is a prerequiste for further visual dysfunction evaluation. If the history suggests color abnormality or color blindness, this can be quantified with Ishihara plates, the Western Aphasia color chart subtest, or the 6-color chart from the Boston Diagnostic Aphasia Test. Commonly employed standard line drawing pictures such as the WAB picture or Boston Aphasia Diagnostic Cookie Theft Picture Test may be used for simultanagnosia testing [33]. Visual form agnosia and associative visual agnosia can be tested by having the person copy drawings of simple objects. These will be deficient in those who have visual form agnosia but not patients who have associative visual agnosia. Associative visual agnosia is tested by demonstrating that identification of an object can be done via other sensory modalities such as auditory or tactile routes. The Boston Naming test (cueing option) can be used to differentiate a naming impairment of an object from visual associative agnosia.

In summary, commonly employed bedside tests include the following:

1. Visual acuity by Snellen or similar chart
2. Visual field testing by confrontation or computerized charting
3. Boston Naming Test
4. Ishihara Plates
5. Line drawings
6. Objects and color identification

A short but yet comprehensive clinical assessment can be made using the subsection of the Coconuts (Chap. 5).

Ventral Occipitotemporal Network for Object and Face Recognition

Complex Visual Processing

Object agnosia: Cannot name 3 objects by visual inspection, but can by touch or sound /3

Achromatopsia: Cannot distinguish 2 different hues or colors. Score 1 for each error /2

Simultanagnosia: CTPT, identify all 3 persons (score 3) or analog time telling (m/h/sec) /3

Optic ataxia: Touch examiners finger under visual guidance. Score 1 for a miss /1

Optic apraxia: Look left, right, up, or down to command. Score 1 for any error /1

Prosopagnosia: Does not recognize family or friends by visual appearance. Score 1 /1

Line orientation: Draw 45-degree and 30-degree lines. Match 2 lines to figure.

Score 1 for each error /2
Subjective report of impaired motion perception (akinetopsia): Score 1 if present /1
Subjective report of depth perception impairment (astereopsis): Score 1 if present /1
Hallucinations: Simple (colors, shapes), complex (scenes, people, animals) or experiential (out of body experience or autoscopy). Score 1 if present /1
Illusions of shape or size: Score 1 if present. For example, macropsia or micropsia /1
Denial of cortical blindness (Anton's syndrome): Score 1 if present /1
Total score: 0 (normal)

Metric Tests

A selection of metric tests helpful for discerning complex visual disorders and their associated hodological syndromes is listed below.

1. Visual Object and Space Perception battery (VOSP)
2. Poppelreuter Overlapping Figures Test
3. Hooper Visual Organization Test
4. Gollin Figures Test
5. Pyramid and Palms Test
6. Birmingham Object Recognition Battery
7. Benton's Judgment of Line Orientation Test
8. Test of Facial Recognition – Famous faces
9. Familiar and unfamiliar faces tests such as the Benton and Van Allen's facial recognition test can be employed for objective assessment
10. Color – Farnsworth's Dichotomous Test for Color Blindness (D-15)
11. Color to Figure Matching Test [34–46]

References

1. Zimmerman M. The nervous system in the context of information theory. In: Schmidt RF, Thews G, editors. Human physiology. Berlin: Springer; 1989. p. 166–73.
2. Hassin RR, Uleman JS, Bargh JA. The new unconscious. Oxford: Oxford University Press; 2006.
3. Rizzo M, Nawrot M, Zihl J. Motion and shape perception in cerebral akinetopsia. Brain. 1995;118:1105–27.
4. Pitzalis S, Sereno MI, Committeri G, Fattori P, Galati G, Tosoni A, Galletti C. The human homologue of macaque area V6A. NeuroImage. 2013;82:517–30.
5. Galletti C, Fattori P, Gamberini M, Kutz DF. The cortical visual area V6: brain location and visual topography. Eur J Neurosci. 1999;11:3922–36.
6. Swisher JD, Halko MA, Merabet LB, McMains SA, Somers DC. Visual topography of human intraparietal sulcus. J Neurosci. 2007;27(20):5326–37.
7. Hadjikhani N, Liu AK, Dale AM, Cavanagh P, Tootell RB. Retinotopy and color sensitivity in human visual cortical area V8. Nat Neurosci. 1998;1(3):235–41.
8. Kandel ER, Schwartz JH, Jessell TM, Siegelbaum SA, Hudspeth AJ, editors. Principles of neural science. 5th ed. McGraw Hill: New York; 2013.

9. Kinsbourne M, Warrington EK. The localizing significance of limited simultaneous visual form perception. Brain. 1963;86:697–702.

10. Hartmann JA, Wolz WA, Roeltgen DP, et al. Denial of visual perception. Brain Cogn. 1991;16:29–40.

11. Zeki S, Ffytche DH. The Riddoch syndrome: insights into the neurobiology of conscious vision. Brain. 1998;121:25–45.

12. Riddoch G. Dissociation of visual perceptions due to occipital injuries, with especial reference to appreciation of movement. Brain. 1917;40:15–57.

13. Wapner W, Judd T, Gardner H. Visual agnosia in an artist. Cortex. 1978;14:343–64.

14. Ffytche D, Blom JD, Catani M. Disorders of visual perception. Neurol Neurosurg Psychiatry. 2010;81:1280e1287. https://doi.org/10.1136/jnnp.2008.171348.

15. Critchley M. The parietal lobes. New York: Hafner Press/MacMillan Publishing Co; 1953.

16. Uchiyama M, Nishio Y, Yokoi K, et al. Pareidolias: complex visual illusions in dementia with Lewy bodies. Brain. 2012;135:2458–69.

17. Michel F, Henaff MA. Seeing without the occipito-parietal cortex: simultanagnosia as a shrinkage of the attentional visual field. Behav Neurol. 2004;15:3–13.

18. Thomas C, Kveraga K, Huberle E, Karnath HO, Bar M. Enabling global processing in simultanagnosia by psychophysical biasing of visual pathways. Brain. 2012;135:1578–85.

19. Whiteside TC, Graybiel A, Niven JI. Visual illusions of movement. Brain. 1965;88:193–210.

20. Kolev OI. Visual hallucinations evoked by caloric vestibular stimulation in normal humans. J Vestib Res. 1995;5:19–23.

21. Uchida H, Suzuki T, Tanaka KF, et al. Recurrent episodes of perceptual alteration in patients treated with antipsychotic agents. J Clin Psychopharmacol. 2003;23:496–9.

22. Battelli L, Pascual-Leone A, Cavanagh P. The 'when' pathway of the right parietal lobe. Trends Cogn Sci. 2007;11:204–10.

23. Mauk MD, Buonomano DV. The neural basis of temporal processing. Annu Rev Neurosci. 2004;27:307–40.

24. Nieder A, Diester I, Tudusciuc O. Temporal and spatial enumeration processes in the primate parietal cortex. Science. 2006;313:1431–5.

25. Bonnet L, Comte A, Tatu L, Millot JL, Moulin T, Medeiros de Bustos E. The role of the amygdala in the perception of positive emotions: an "intensity detector" Front Behav Neurosci 2015;9:178. doi: https://doi.org/10.3389/fnbeh.2015.00178. eCollection 2015.

26. Benarroch EE. The amygdala: functional organization and involvement in neurologic disorders. Neurology. 2015;84(3):313–24.

27. Critchley M. Metamorphopsia of central origin. Trans Ophthalmol Soc UK. 1949;69:111–21.

28. Ellis HD, Young AW, Quayle AH, De Pauw KW. Reduced autonomic responses to faces in Capgras delusion. Proc Biol Sci. 1997;264:1085–92.

29. Bischof M, Bassetti CL. Total dream loss: a distinct neuropsychological dysfunction after bilateral PCA stroke. Ann Neurol. 2004;56:583–6.

30. Peña-Casanova J, Roig-Rovira T, Bermudez A, Tolosa-Sarro E. Optic aphasia, optic apraxia, and loss of dreaming. Brain Lang. 1985;26(1):63–71.

31. Santos-Bueso E, Serrador-Garcia M, Porta-Etessam J, et al. Charles Bonnet syndrome. A 45 case series. Rev Neurol. 2015;60:337–40.

32. Benke T. Peduncular hallucinosis – a syndrome of impaired reality monitoring. J Neurol. 2006;253:1561–71.

33. Beck DM, Rees G, Frith CD, Lavie N. Neural correlates of change and change blindness. Nat Neurosci. 2001;4:645–50.

34. Rock I, Linnet CM, Grant PI, Mack A. Perception without attention: results of a new method. Cogn Psychol. 1992;24:502–34.

35. Scholte HS, Witteveen SC, Spekreijse H, Lamme VA. The influence of inattention on the neural correlates of scene segmentation. Brain Res. 2006;1076:106–15.

36. Windmann S, Wehrmann M, Calabrese P, Gunturkun O. Role of the prefrontal cortex in attentional control over bistable vision. J Cogn Neurosci. 2006;18:456–71.

37. Frith CD. In: Kandel ER, Schwartz JH, editors. Principles of neural science. 5th ed. New York: McGraw Hill; 2013.
38. Hoffmann M, Keiseb J, Moodley J, Corr P. Appropriate neurological evaluation and multimodality magnetic resonance imaging in eclampsia. Acta Neurol Scand. 2002;106(3):159–67.
39. Lezak MD, Howieson DB, Bigler ED, Tranel T, editors. Neuropsychological assessment. Oxford: Oxford University Press; 2012.
40. Warrington E, James M. VOSP. Harcourt assessment. The psychological corporation. London: The Thames Valley Test Company; 1991.
41. Brandt J. The Hopkins verbal learning test: development of a new memory test with six equivalent forms. Clin Neuropsychol. 1991;5:125–42.
42. Randolph C. Manual: repeatable battery for the assessment of neuropsychological status. San Antonio: Psychological Corporation; 1998.
43. Hodges JR, Salmon DP, Butters N. Recognition and naming of famous faces in Alzheimer's disease: a cognitive analysis. Neuropsychologia. 1993;31:775–88.
44. Osterrieth PA. Le test de copie d'une figure complexe. Archive de Psychologie. 1944;30:206–356 and L'examen RA. Psychologique dans les cas d'encephalopathie traumatique. Archives de Psychologie. 1941;28:286–340.
45. Boston Naming Test, Kaplan E, Goodglass H, Weintraub S. Boston naming test. 2nd ed. Boston: Lippincott Williams & Wilkins; 2001.
46. Howard D, Patterson K. Pyramids and palm trees: a test of semantic access from pictures and words. Bury St Edmunds: Thames Valley Test Company; 1992.
47. Barrett KE, Barman SM, Boitano S, Brooks HL, editors. Ganong's review of medical physiology. 25th ed. New York: McGraw Hill; 2016.
48. Smith SM, Fox PT, Miller KL, et al. Correspondence of the brain's functional architecture during activation and rest. PNAS. 2009;106:13040–5.
49. Catani M, Jones DK, Donato R, Ffytche DH. Occipito-temporal connections in the human brain. Brain. 2003;126:2093–107.
50. Caverzasi E, Papinutto N, Amirbekian B, Berger MS, Henry RG. Q-ball of inferior Frontooccipital fasciculus and beyond. PLoS One. 2014;9(6):e100274.

Chapter 12
Provincial Hub Syndromes, Temporal, Parietal and Acquired Cultural Circuit Syndromes

At times, more restricted lesions of the brain areas may lead to involvement of so-called provincial hubs or more localized or confined brain regions. Several typical brain images are presented in Fig. 12.1. The parietal and temporal lobes are often involved with such lesions and both have been reported as relatively "silent" areas of the brain when restricted lesions affect these areas. A case in point is that of image 1 in figure. The middle-aged woman presented as a so-called "stroke alert" to our emergency room with her main presenting symptom a sudden severe headache with otherwise normal neurological examination and normal NIH stroke score of 0. With administration of analgesics, a rapid improvement of her headache ensued and she was cleared for discharge with a presumptive diagnosis of migraine to which she was prone to. Just prior to her discharge, the fasttracked MRI scan became available and revealed a small left parietal hemorrhage. Given the location, she was evaluated for left parietal syndromes including a Gerstmann's syndrome and angular gyrus syndrome, the former which was her ultimate clinical diagnosis. In emergent as well as most routine stroke presentations, Gerstmann's syndrome is rarely specifically tested for, and indeed in our case it was the only discernible neurological deficit. This brief case report underscores the value of cognitive and behavioral neurological syndrome evaluation. In emergent cases, neuroimaging is often revealing and can guide the examination. Given a lesion, what specific syndromes may be present?

The parietal and temporal lobes may be involved in isolation, at times only involving a gyrus or only the precuneus or claustrum by discrete lesions caused by stroke, amyloid angiopathy, tumors, and even parietal or temporal lobe seizures (Fig. 12.1). Many of the syndromes will present with the so-called acquired cultural circuitry and appear as syndromes of apraxia, alexia, acalculia, agraphia, amusia, and art. However, some, such as the reading and praxis circuits, are much more distributed with wide ranging networks (Fig. 12.2). Emotion disorders are primarily a temporal lobe function, and even though the brain's emotional circuitry is extensive and widespread involving many cortical and subcortical regions, the temporal lobe serves as an important hub. A list of potential syndromes is presented according to basic anatomical (or provincial hub) areas.

© Springer Nature Switzerland AG 2020
M. Hoffmann, *Clinical Mentation Evaluation*,
https://doi.org/10.1007/978-3-030-46324-3_12

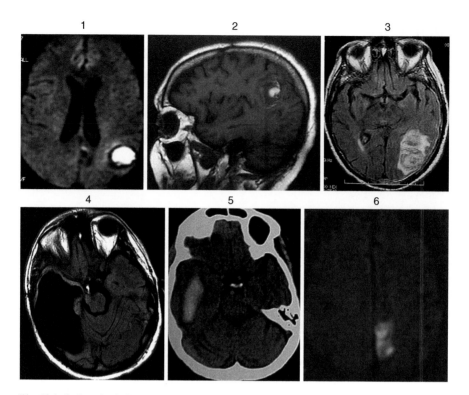

Fig. 12.1 Left parietal, discrete, amyloid angiopathy-related hemorrhage with sole clinical deficit; Gerstmann's syndrome (1). Ideomotor apraxia in a patient with a small left inferior parietal hemorrhage (2). Alexia without agraphia due to left occipitoparietal hemorrhage (3). Right temperoparietal post-traumatic lesion presenting with amusia (4). Right temporal hemorrhage manifesting with Gastaut-Geschwind syndrome (5). Precuneus infarct with obtundation due to distal thrombosis of anterior cerebral artery callosomarginal branch occlusion (6)

Right or Left Parietal Lesions Syndromes

Syndromes of Cortical Sensory Impairment

1. Astereognosis – loss of depth perception
2. Two-point discrimination impairment
3. Agraphesthesia – palm number tracing impairment
4. Abaragnosia – loss of weight perception discrimination
5. Tactile agnosia – able to describe precisely the size, shape, contour, and position of an object, but unable to recognize what the object is or what function it may have

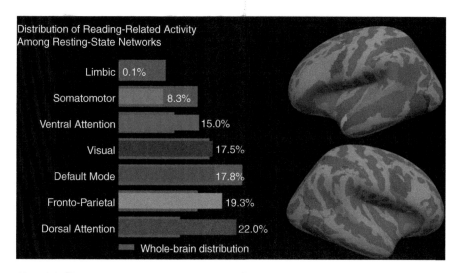

Fig. 12.2 Visual, default mode, and cingulo-opercular networks required for reading skill. Reading areas are distributed across several networks with attention and executive networks particularly important and hubs including the inferior frontal gyrus and temporoparietal junction. (Figure with permission Baily et al. [28])

6. Ahylognosia – inability to distinguish texture of objects
7. Parietal pain syndromes – the parietal operculum (BA 43) is also referred to as the secondary somatosensory cortex (SII). The SII and the posterior insular region are essential for normal pain and tactile perception. Tumors or seizures of these regions may be associated with a contralateral hemi-body, burning-type pain syndrome

Visuospatial Dysfunction Syndromes

1. Balint's syndrome – simultanagnosia, visual apraxia, visual ataxia
2. Optokinetic reflex and optokinetic nystagmus (OKN), smooth pursuit/saccadic eye movement disorders

Temporo-occipito-parietal (TOP) Junction Functions and Other Cross Modal Sensory Abnormalities

1. Autoscopy – seeing one's double often from a vantage point also referred to as an out of body experience

2. Acquired synesthesia – cross modal sensory experiences whereby a sensory stimulus of one modality triggers sensations in another modality. Color grapheme is most common
3. Cotard's syndrome – denial of existence, a perceptual emotional derangement [1]
4. Migraine phenomena – autokinesis (apparent movement of objects in the dark), inversion of two- and three-dimensional vision, body weight, and size perception disturbance [2]

Attention and Consciousness Hubs (Precuneus and Claustrum)

1. Minimally conscious states
2. Anesthesia
3. Transcendental states

Miscellaneous Conditions

1. Parietal arm levitation – outstretched hands, spontaneous contralateral arm elevation [3]
2. Poikilotonia – erratic and variable tone alteration from hypotonia to hypertonia [3]
3. Parietal avoidance syndrome [4]
4. Parietal wasting syndrome – rare occurrence of wasting of contralateral arm or leg attributed to parietal lobe lesions [5]
5. Pain processing in parietal lobes and phantom limb pain [6]
6. Algodiaphoria – indifference to painful stimuli
7. Parietal seizures
8. Conversion disorders

Left Parietal Lesions: Typically

1. Anomias – word production, word selection, semantic
2. Apraxias – ideomotor, melokinetic
3. Gerstmann's syndrome – acalculia, agraphia, R/L orientation, finger anomia
4. Angular gyrus syndrome – features of Gerstmann's plus alexia and anomia
5. Autotopagnosia – inability to name or localize body parts (inferior parietal)

Right Parietal Lesions: Typically

1. Visuoconstructive impairment
2. Visuospatial impairment
3. Aprosodias – alteration in melodic intonation of speech, expressive or receptive types
4. Neglect syndromes
5. Anosognosias and related syndromes – denial or underestimation of weakness
6. Geographic disorientation
7. Allesthesias – transference of sensation from the impaired limb to the opposite intact limb
8. Aphonognosia – unable to recognize familiar voices, akin to the visual impairment, prosopagnosia [7, 8]
9. Dressing apraxia
10. Event timing
11. Perception of sound movements [9]
12. Three-dimensional sense appreciation impairment

Bedside and Metric Testing

Coconuts subtests for the following:

• Language- and praxis-related tests if left hemisphere implicated
• Visuospatial tests for right hemisphere lesions

Parietal basic and multimodality processing capabilities test for the following:

1. Basic sensory – tactile, vibration, pain
2. Cortical sensory abilities – 2-point discrimination, graphesthesia, barognosis
3. Optokinetic nystagmus – use rotating drum or strip of alternating colors
4. Interlocking finger test [10]
5. Cross modal testing by the bouba Kiki phenomenon – the mapping of vocal sounds to the visual features of a specific object being related and non-arbitrary [11, 12]
6. Synesthesia (multimodal processing) – inquire after number–color associations, for example

Metric Tests for Inferior Parietal Lobe Abilities

1. Boston Naming Test (BNT) to assess for anomias – words are multimodality (parietal) symbols for ideas, objects

2. Using the cueing option of the BNT, a differentiation between anomias and semantic memory loss (anterior temporal lobe) may be made
3. Metaphors testing. This can be tested, for example, by the proverb sub-test of the DKEFS which provides a scoring system and normative data. DKEFS proverbs include [13] the following.

Superior Parietal Lobe Function Test

1. Praxis testing and the apraxia deficits are depicted below

Alexias

Alexia syndrome denotes the acquired inability to read, despite intact elementary anterior visual function such as acuity, and neurologically intact object and color identification. Most lesions usually involve the left occipital region resulting in a right homonymous hemianopia and reading impairment. At times, these patients may perform what is termed letter by letter reading characterized by slow and laborious reading output. Alexias may be classified into peripheral and central subtypes.

Peripheral

1. Alexia with agraphia
2. Alexia without agraphia
3. Frontal alexia (third alexia) – the reading impairment that occurs with Broca's aphasia
4. Hemialexia – can read only the right half of a word due to corpus callosal lesions interrupting fibers crossing from the RH with left hemifield vision impairment
5. Spatial alexia – occurs in association with left field visual neglect syndrome (RH lesions). More complex words such as "workplace" may be read instead as "place"

Central Deep Alexia (Paralexia)

1. Paralexia (deep dyslexia) – the substitution of content-related words during reading, for example boat for ship

Increased Function

1. Hyperlexia – a compulsion to read aloud verbage in their immediate environment including labels, warning, traffic signs

Congenital

1. Dyslexia

Agraphia Classification

Writing is an acquired higher cortical function ability that straddles both language
and praxis abilities and impairments may be recognized with aphasias or apraxias
as a consequence. Agraphia is frequent with aphasia, particularly with the expressive dysphasia. In addition, several other forms of agraphic syndromes may be
recognized.

Primary Agraphia

1. Pure isolated agraphia – associated with alexia but no apraxia or aphasia. Occurs
   with left posterior frontal lesions (Exner's area) or less often with superior left
   parietal
2. Central (aphasic) agraphia – similar to aphasia, may be non-fluent, phonological,
   lexical, or semantic
3. Deep agraphia – lesions affect both phonological ability and orthographic memory and cannot recall how words look with correct spelling, nor sound them out.
   Lesions are in the left parietal region

Secondary Agraphia

1. Aphasic agraphia
2. Apractic agraphia
3. Visuospatial agraphia
4. Micrographia
5. Paretic agraphia – related to peripheral nerve or myopathic process

Other Variants

1. Hypergraphia – may occur with right hemisphere lesions or Gastaut-Geschwind syndrome
2. Dystypia – isolated-type impairments without aphasia, apraxia, or even agraphia with lesions in the second left frontal gyrus and adjacent frontal operculum

Anarithmetria and Acalculias

The underlying cause may be primary such as anarithmetria or secondary such as aphasia, alexia, or visuospatial dysfunction. The four basic arithmetic functions are represented in different brain areas, mostly elucidated by functional imaging brain activation studies:

- Subtraction – bilateral intraparietal activation
- Multiplication – posterior and left angular gyrus activity
- Addition – left anterior inferior frontal Broca's and angular gyrus regions
- Approximation of quantity dependent on the bilateral intraparietal sulci

Primary

1. Transcoding impairment – correct digit reproduction but misplaced in the order of magnitude, for example one hundred and 50 is transcribed as 10050
2. Asymbolic acalculia – disability of interpretation of operation symbols such as multiplication, division, addition, or subtraction
3. Selective anarithmetria – selective calculation impairment seen with left parietal damage. For example, may be good with subtraction and addition but unable to perform division or multiplication procedures

Secondary

1. Aphasic dyscalculia
2. Visuospatial dyscalculia
3. Alexic dyscalculia
4. Inattention dyscalclulia

Bedside Testing

- Serial 7's testing
- Doubling in 2's or 3's

Metric Testing

- WAIS-IV calculation subtests
- DKEFS calculation subtests

Apraxias

The term apraxia applies to the syndromes of inability to perform skilled motor acts in the context of normal or near-normal elementary neurological function of sensation and motor power. There should also be adequate domains of attention and no significant cognitive or movement disorders. Apraxias are more common in the context of aphasia, occurring in over half of these patients, and constitute one of several neurological syndromes whereby the impairment is not volunteered by patients. Apraxias are important to diagnose as they have a significant effect on the rehabilitation success, are usually associated with left hemisphere pathology, and may occur separate from aphasias.

Classification of Apraxias

Limb

1. Ideomotor – may be due to postural errors, the incorrect joint, incorrect targeting of the intended object, or using body part as tool error (the hand or fingers are used as the tool). The main hub area is the left supramarginal gyrus
2. Melokinetic – a relatively mild form of apraxia with impairment of the deftness of finger and hand movements. Also termed limb kinetic dyspraxia
3. Sympathetic – an ideomotor apraxia may affect both hands, which is due to lesions in the white matter adjacent to Broca's area in the left hemisphere disconnecting the two motor association areas of the hemispheres

4. Conduction – the imitation of learned transitive movements are more impaired than pantomiming the same movements. People with ideomotor generally imitate transitive gestures better than pantomiming transitive gestures to verbal instruction
5. Conceptual – refers to the loss of the specific mechanical knowledge of a tool or an implement and may include tool selection deficit, tool action association deficit
6. Verbal motor dissociation – failure to execute gestures in response to visual input, but correctly perform verbal instruction
7. Tactile motor dissociation apraxia – tactile exploration of shapes impaired with a dissociation in shape recognition using either active and passive touch. A pure tactile apraxia without tactile agnosia
8. Pantomime agnosia – a deficiency in the tactile object recognition due to an impairment of recognizing object shape, despite normal sensorimotor functions. The fault may be with loss of integrated exploratory hand movements

Axial

1. Axial apraxia – difficulties of abnormal postures turning over while recumbent, arising from supine or sitting position, often seen in Parkinson's and progressive supranuclear palsy

Buccofacial

1. Oral apraxia – difficulty with performing skilled movements of the lips, tongue, face, pharynx, and larynx

Complex (Frontal Lobe Based)

1. Ideational apraxia – impairment in performing multistep (3 or more) sequential actions to command
2. Ideomotor prosodic apraxia – normal prosody during spontaneous speech but unable to produce specific acoustical variations to verbal command

Task Specific

1. Gait apraxia – at times taking the form of gait ignition failure presenting with hesitation in starting to walk and in turning, not associated with elementary neurological impairment such as motor, sensory, or cerebellar deficits
2. Ocular apraxia – impaired gaze direction to command. This may be a component of Balint's syndrome

3. Apraxia of eyelid opening – after RH infarction, patients remain with eyes closed, unable to open them to command, but they may spontaneously open their eyes
4. Dressing apraxia – lacking intact visuospatial functioning with typical examples referring to putting on a shirt on back to front, or inside out
5. Constructional apraxia – an impairment in drawing, assembling, or building, without there being an apraxia for single movements
6. Apraxic agraphia – slow, effortful, imprecise letter formation with distortions which result in illegible handwriting

Bedside Testing

1. Ideomotor limb Intransitive

Arm
Wave goodbye
Beckon, come here
Leg
Place one foot in front of the other as if tandem walking
Describe a circle with the foo

2. Ideomotor limb transitive

Arm
Pretend to use a pair of scissors cutting a piece of paper
Pretend to use a toothbrush, brushing your teeth
Leg
Kick a ball
Pretend to accelerate by pushing on a gas pedal

3. Buccofacial

Whistle
Pretend to blow out a candle

4. Axial

Stand like a boxer
Stand like a golfer getting ready to swing
Bend the head forward and backward
Shrug or lift both shoulders

5. Melokinetic

Rapid opposition of the thumb to each of the four fingers forward and backward
Compare right to left hand

6. Ideational

Write your address on a piece of paper, fold it in half, and place inside a book
  or folder
Coconuts subtest for apraxia (Chap. 5)

Metric Tests

- Brief Apraxia Screening Test [14]
- STIMA test [15]
- Van Heugten Test for Apraxia [16]
- Short Apraxia Screening Test [17]
- Florida Apraxia Battery [18]
- TULIA Test [19]

Temporal Lobe Cognitive and Behavioral Syndromes

The temporal lobes are extensively connected to the other cerebral lobes via association tracts with the occipitotemporal tract the second largest long-range association tracts. The uncinate fasciculus is also a prominent connecting the temporal lobe
with the inferior frontal lobe. Lesions of the anterior temporal lobe, inferior frontal
lobe, and the uncinate fasciculus are commonly implicated together. Because of
both the close association of the uncinate fasciculus with the anterior temporal lobe
and inferior frontal lobe some researchers refer to syndromes in these regions as
uncinate fasciculus syndromes as the most appropriate approach. Sensory visual,
auditory, and olfactory, in approximate order of importance, mediate evaluation of
another person's eye gaze, body movements, facial expressions, tonality and even
nonconsciously perceived sensory stimuli including pheromones. The temporal
lobes play a critical role in societal interaction. Specialized and separate temporal
cortical areas have been identified for these.

Right or Left and Bilateral

Elementary Neurological

1. Vertiginous syndromes – vertigo or disequilibrium due to epilepsy or migraine
2. Olfactory hallucinations due to uncinate lesions or seizures
3. Gustatory (taste) abnormalities due to medial temporal or insula lesions or
   seizures

Neuropsychiatric – anxiety, agitation, paranoia, aggression

Behavioral Neurological

1. Geschwind-Gastaut syndrome – viscous personality, hypergraphia, metaphysical preoccupation
2. Klüver–Bucy syndrome – hyperorality, placidity, visual agnosia, hypermetamorphosis
3. Involuntary emotional expression disorder (IEED)

Social Disorders Associated with Primarily Temporal Lobe Dysfunction

1. Williams syndrome – marked hypersociality, hypermusical, and hypernarrative. These present during childhood with other traits including characteristic facial features of wide mouth, upturned nose, small chin, "starry eyes," cardiac abnormalities, hypercalcemia
2. Urbach-Wiethe disease – social handicap associated with memory impairments
3. Autoimmune encephalitis – neuropsychiatric presentations, a wide variety of temporal lobe syndromes, memory dysfunction, and seizures

Cognitive Neurological

1. Korsakoff amnestic state
2. Cortical deafness
3. Auditory agnosia – inability to identify sounds despite normal peripheral hearing status
4. Auditory paracusias – auditory hallucinations (simple and complex), auditory illusions
5. Chronoataraxis – disorders of time perception (time may pass with excessive speed or very slowly)

Emotional Intelligence (EI)

EI is critical for navigating social complexities and has been correlated with personal success and career achievements [20]. EI deficiencies may be present after traumatic brain injury stroke, multiple sclerosis, and frontotemporal syndromes but may overlap with normalcy and in otherwise healthy people [21, 22]. The EI networks include hubs in anterior cingulate cortex, orbitofrontal cortex, insula, and amygdaloid complex [23, 24]. The 5 principal EI composite factors and 15 subcategories in the Baron EQ-I test include [23] the following:

• Intrapersonal – self-regard, emotional self-awareness, independence, self-actualization

- Interpersonal – empathy, social responsibility, interpersonal relationship
- Stress management – stress tolerance, impulse control
- Adaptability – reality testing, flexibility, problem-solving
- General mood – optimism, happiness

Left Temporal

Elementary Neurological

Right upper quadrantanopia

Cognitive

1. Aphasias – Wernicke's, transcortical sensory and anomic
2. Memory – verbal amnesia
3. Visual agnosia
4. Lexical amusia – impairment in reading music
5. Synesthesia – a sensory stimulus presented in one modality engenders a sensation in another sensory modality. The most common is grapheme color, but over 60 different synesthesia subtypes have been described

Right Temporal

Elementary

1. Left upper quadrantanopia

Cognitive

1. Memory – visuospatial amnesia
2. Prosopagnosia – right anterior temporal lobe
3. Auditory agnosia – verbal (pure word deafness) and non-verbal (environmental sounds)
4. Delusional misidentification syndromes

Amusias

1. Receptive amusia – impairment in appreciating music such as songs
2. Expressive amusia – impairment in singing or playing a musical instrument

3. Instrumental amusia – loss of prior ability to play a musical instrument
4. Musical alexia – acquired inability to read musical notes
5. Musical agraphia – acquired inability to write musical notes
6. Musical amnesia – acquired inability to recall well-known songs and tunes

Temporal Lobe Beside Testing (Coconuts Subtest, Chap. 5)

Hippocampal Limbic Network for Memory and Emotion

Memory: score 1 for each error, 0 is normal
Short-term memory: Register five words (orange, ocean, courage, rapid, building)
Test recall at 5 min. Score 1 for each omission /5
Remote memory: Recite last 3 presidents or 3 important personal dates (graduations) /3

Emotions

Lability: laughs or cries easily, out of context. Rarely (1), sometimes (2), frequently (3), never (0) /3
Geschwind-Gastaut syndrome: Stroke or new lesion induced new evidence of viscous personality, metaphysical pre-occupation, and altered physiological drives

(i) Viscous personality: One or more of the following. Circumstantiality in speech, over-inclusive verbal discourse, excessive detail of information, stickiness of thought processes, interpersonal adhesiveness, prolongation of interpersonal encounters, and hypergraphia

(ii) Metaphysical pre-occupation: One or more of the following: overly philosophical pre-occupation, nascent and excessive intellectual interests in religion, philosophy, and moral issues

(iii) Altered physiological drives: One or more of the following: hyposexuality, aggression, fear

Scoring: 2 out of 3 components required for diagnosis
Score as 3 components (3), 2 components (2), 1 component (1), nil (0) /3

Temporal Lobe Metric Tests

Center for Neurologic Study – Lability Scale for IEED evaluation [25]
Baron EQ-1 – for emotional intelligence [23]
Bear Fedio – for diagnosis of Gastaut-Geschwind syndrome [26]
Montreal Battery for Evaluation of Amusia [27]

References

1. Ramirez-Bermudez J, Aguilar-Venegas LC, Crail-Melendez D, Espinola-Nadurille M, Nente F, Mendez MF. Cotard syndrome in neurological and psychiatric patients. J Neuropsychiatry Clin Neurosci. 2010;22(4):409–16.
2. Jürgens TP, Schulte LH, May A. Migraine trait symptoms in migraine with and without aura. Neurology. 2014;82(16):1416–24.
3. Ghika J, Ghika-Schmid F, Bogousslasvky J. Parietal motor syndrome: a clinical description in 32 patients in the acute phase of pure parietal strokes studied prospectively. Clin Neurol Neurosurg. 1998;100(4):271–82.
4. Critchley M. The parietal lobes. London: Hafner Press/Collier MacMillan Publishers; 1953.
5. Maramattom BV. Parietal wasting and dystonia secondary to a parasagittal mass lesion. Neurol India. 2007;55(2):185.
6. Sandyk R. Spontaneous pain, hyperpathia and wasting of the hand due to parietal lobe haemorrhage. Eur Neurol. 1985;24:1–3.
7. Van Lancker DR, Kreiman J, Cummings J. Voice perception deficits: neuroanatomical correlates of phonagnosia. J Clin Exp Neuropsychol. 1989;11(5):665–74.
8. Biederman I, Herald S, Xu X, Amir O, Shilowich B. Phonagnosia, a Voice Homologue to Prosopagnosia. J Vis. 2015;15(12):1206. https://doi.org/10.1167/15.12.1206.
9. Griffiths TD, Rees G, Tees A, Green GRA, Witton C, Rowe D, Buechel C, Turner R, Frackowiak RSJ. Right parietal lobe is involved in the perception of sound movements in humans. Nat Neurosci. 1998;1:74–9.
10. Moo LR, Slotnick SD, Tesoro MA, Zee DS, Hart J. Interlocking finger test: a bedside screen for parietal lobe dysfunction. J Neurol Neurosurg Psychiatry. 2003;74(4):530–2.
11. Köhler W. Gestalt psychology. New York: Liveright; 1929.
12. Ramachandran VS, Hubbard EM. Synaesthesia: a window into perception, thought and language. J Conscious Stud. 2001;8:3–34.
13. Delis DC, Kaplan E, Kramer JH, Delis D. Kaplan executive function system. San Antonio: Pearson; 2001.
14. Efros DB, Cimino-Knight AM, Morelli CA, et al. A comparison of two assessment methods for ideomotor limb apraxia. San Diego: American Speech Language Hearing Association Annual Convention; 2005.
15. Tessari A, Toraldo A, Lunardelli A, et al. STIMA: a short screening test for ideo-motor apraxia, selective for action meaning and bodily district. Neurol Sci. 2015;36:977–84.
16. Smits L, Flapper M, Sistermans N, et al. Apraxia in mild cognitive impairment and Alzheimer's disease: validity and reliability of the Van Heugten test for apraxia. Dement Geriatr Cogn Disord. 2014;38:55–64.
17. Leiguarda R, Clarens F, Amengual A, Drucaroff L, Hallett M. Short apraxia screening test. J Clin Exp Neuropsychol. 2014;36(8):867–74. https://doi.org/10.1080/13803395.2014.951315.
18. Power E, Code C, Croot K, Sheard C. Florida Apraxia Battery–Extended and Revised Sydney (FABERS): Design, description, and a healthy control sampleJournal of Clinical and Experimental Neuropsychology 2009;32(1):1–18.
19. Vanbellingen T, Kersten B, Van Hemelrijk B, Van de Winckel A, Bertschi M, Müri R, De Weerdt W, Bohlhalter S. Comprehensive assessment of gesture production: a new test of upper limb apraxia (TULIA). Eur J Neurol. 2010;17(1):59–66.
20. Goleman DP. Emotional intelligence: why it can matter more than IQ for character, health and lifelong achievement. New York: Bantam Books; 1995.
21. Mendez MF, Lauterbach EC, Sampson SM. An evidence-based review of the psychopathology of frontotemporal dementia: a report of the ANPA committee16 on research. J Neuropsychiatry Clin Neurosci. 2008;20(2):130–49.
22. Van der Zee J, Sleegers K, Van Broeckhoven C. The Alzheimer disease frontotemporal lobar degeneration spectrum. Neurology. 2008;71:1191–7.

23. Bar-On R, Tranel D, Denburg NL, Bechara A. Exploring the neurological substrate of emotional and social intelligence. Brain. 2003;126:1790–800.

24. Shamay-Tsoory SG, Tomer R, Goldsher D, Berger BD, Aharon-Peretz J. Impairment in cognitive and affective empathy in patients with brain lesions:anatomical and cognitive correlates. J Clin Exp Neuropsychol. 2004;26(8):1113–27.

25. Lauterbach EC, Cummings JL, Kuppuswamy PS. Toward a more precise, clinically – informed pathophysiology of pathological laughing and crying. Neurosci Biobehav Rev. 2013;37(8):1893–916.

26. Bear DM, Fedio P. Quantitative analysis of interictal behavior in temporal lobe epilepsy. Arch Neurol. 1977;34:454.

27. Peretz I, Champod S, Hyde K. Varieties of musical disorders: the Montreal battery of evaluation of Amusia. Ann N Y Acad Sci. 2003;999:58–75.

28. Baily SK, Aboud KS, Nguyen TQ, Cutting LE. Applying a network framework to the neurobiology of reading and dyslexia. J Neurodev Disord. 2018;10:37. https://doi.org/10.1186/s11689-018-9251-z.

Chapter 13
Neuroplasticity and Other Treatment Options for Cognitive and Behavioral Neurological Syndromes

It would be a remiss not to have a section enunciating potential treatments of the several hundred cognitive and behavioral syndromes mentioned in the foregoing chapters. There has been renewed focus on working with the brain's inherent neuroplasticity, which has been relatively ignored until recently. The predominant focus over the past few decades has been on neuropharmacological or pill-centric approaches. Furthermore, we have also had a gene-centric approach that had been initially promising since the recently completed Human Genome Project. This too has given way to the epigenetic and small RNA science from direct environmental influences. Finally, due to a memory-centric culture over the past few decades, much of clinical dementia and mild cognitive impairment may have been obscured by other important symptoms and dementias other than Alzheimer's disease.

Neuropharmacological management remains the mainstay of psychiatry treatment options, primarily targeting the ascending neurotransmitter modulatory systems. However, these are only one of many widely distributed brain network systems and are intrinsically nonspecific and hence limited in their benefits for people with neuropsychiatric syndromes. Approaches that target the underlying cause with more enduring outcome are therapies involving the manipulation of the brain's own neuroplasticity. This type of brain training is particularly appealing because of the notion of generalization and transfer effect. For example, a brain training program may enhance one particular skill, but the effects are relegated to other areas and so may ramify widely to other brain circuitries. This "transfer effect" that may convey a more general improvement in cognitive performance, may transmit to other cognitive functions. The specific plastic changes in the motor and sensory networks at the molecular substrate, take the form of rapid dendritic spine formation as well as redundant spine elimination during sleep.

Prior to using general and specific target therapies for augmenting brain function, the principal of a fit body translating into a fit mind requires emphasis. A profusion of clinical studies now point to physical exercise and correct nutrition as being not only disease-modifying therapies, but they can also dramatically reduce the incidence of stroke, dementia, and cognitive decline. Not only do physical exercise and cognitive training build new gray and white matter, but meditation also may facilitate specific prefrontal neurogenesis and white matter proliferation that have been shown to ameliorate some of our most challenging conditions such as PTSD and depression. More specific interventions (devices, drugs, surgery) may then enable advantageous targeted stimulation, or inhibition of different circuits, or a combination of both to boost brain function.

A quinary focus should take the form of the following:

1. Disease mechanism elucidation, bolstered by connectomic understanding
2. Optimizing vascular and neuronal health through the 5 brain fitness rules
3. Focused therapies taking a renewed emphasis on neuroplastic treatment mechanisms
4. Microbiome health and attention to senotherapeutics
5. Neuropharmacological therapies where these have unequivocally shown to be of value

Without precise diagnosis or at least a comprehensive differential diagnosis where the presentation defies precise characterization, treatment strategies are destined to fail or may even worsen the patient. Allied to this premise, the deliberate search for medications causing side effects and adding to the underlying impairment, is often of benefit. A good example is the anticholinergic effect present in many of the major drug groups, that can aggravate a memory disorder or acute confusional state. Once a treatment plan has been formulated, both pharmacotherapy and augmenting the supporting mechanisms of spontaneous recovery, are key.

Identify and intervene early on in the process of vascular inflammation that leads to cognitive vascular disorder and neurodegeneration. This chronic, smoldering process of vascular inflammation leads to cognitive impairment over years or decades. The timely advocation of physical exercise, which exerts powerful anti-inflammatory effects, into brain treatment protocols is advocated. The daily formation and dismantling of neuronal assemblies constitute a normal part of the brain's activity. Recently, the importance of sleep has surged with the realization that off-line synaptic pruning and cerebral glymphatics or "brain-washing" are fundamental functions in eliminating neurotoxic waste that accumulates in the waking state, underlying the restorative function of sleep [1].

Whereas pharmacotherapy targets mainly the ascending monoaminergic systems, neuroplasticity approaches such as cognitive behavioral therapy deploy the top-down influence of the prefrontal cortex. Some lesions have both excitatory and inhibitory influences on different brain networks and even hemisphere. Aphasia is a good example that can be treated by transcranial magnetic stimulation which can both increase activity the affected left hemisphere with excitatory influences with high frequency repetitive TMS or dampen the excitatory influences of the unaffected right hemisphere by inhibitory low frequency settings (Fig. 13.1) [2]. Mirror visual feedback therapy that has been used to alleviate phantom limb pain, for instance, is another good example (Fig. 13.2).

Neuroplasticity refers to the brain's inherent capacity to respond to environmental demands consisting of both white and gray matter structural changes in the motor and sensory cortical regions mediated by or marked by expeditious new dendritic

Fig. 13.1 transcranial magnetic stimulation(TMS) and transcranial direct current stimulation (tDCS). (Fregni and Pascual-Leone [2])

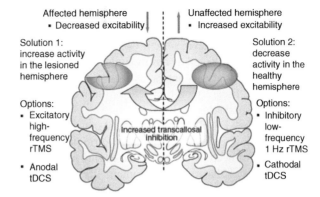

Fig. 13.2 Using mirror neurons to heal. Mirror therapy for phantom limb pain treatment. Ramachandran and Altschuler [83]. The use of visual feedback, in particular mirror visual feedback, in restoring brain function

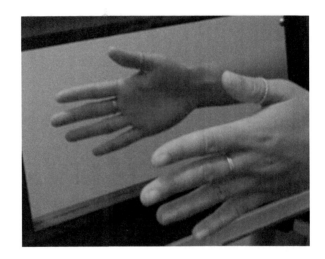

spine formation. An appreciation of the rapidity of effects that may be seen with some of these interventions, for example, grey matter volume increases occurred:

- After several days of signature writing using the non-dominant hand
- Within 2 weeks of practicing mirror reading
- Over the course of several months of practicing juggling

In addition, plastic changes were also engendered by becoming proficient in a foreign language, with training in a spatial navigation program and playing video games. The training augments the particular competence being practiced, and the proposed concept of generalization and transfer posits that enhancement may be transmitted to other cognitive abilities. Improving working memory, for example, by computerized programs has been shown to improve other cognitive abilities such as executive function [3, 4].

Practicing a particular skill through intensive training is specific for that skill. Other neuroplasticity enhancements such as physical exercise have more general-ized effects on overall cognition including speed of information processing mediated by neural growth factor release such as BDNF and increased vascularization. Executive function has been shown to improve in young middle-aged adults (aged 20–67) engaged in aerobic exercise, for example, after 24 weeks [5]. Physical exercise is being touted as a fifth vital sign, and consequently is important to measure in all clinical encounters, as well as when engaging in various preventative therapies or disease-modifying therapy for mild cognitive impairment, dementia, brain aging, and stroke [6].

The Finnish FINGER study reported that employing a multidomain intervention of physical exercise, appropriate nutrition, cognitive stimulation, and self-monitoring of heart health prevented cognitive decline in at-risk older adults. It has been estimated that this multidomain lifestyle intervention can achieve a 25% reduction in Alzheimer's disease [7]. The FINGER model is now being adapted in US POINTER study, Asia SINGER study, China MIND-CHINA study, Australia MYB study, and Europe MIND-AD study.

Wave Therapy and Neurostimulation

Inducing specific wave therapies may hold promise for combating neurodegenerative diseases. A groundbreaking study by Hughes et al. in people with frontotemporal lobar degeneration (FTD) noted a reduction in beta resynchronization with a concomitant reorganization of interregional connectivity together with an elevation of gamma coupling between the motor cortex and pre-supplementary motor area (pre-SMA). It has been postulated that the loss of oscillatory power in certain neurodegenerative diseases is a neurobiological disease mechanism accounting for behavioral disinhibition leading to clinically appreciated disinhibited behavior and inappropriate actions [8].

There is accruing evidence for Alzheimer's, schizophrenia, and Parkinson's treatment with such therapies including reversal of the process [9]. Acoustic therapies such as "pink noise" (waterfall sound) when administered to sleeping adults caused an increase in the amplitude of slow waves which was associated with a 25–30% improvement in recalling words learnt during the previous night [10]. From animal studies, we have learnt that gamma oscillations (25–140 Hz) in area of mice brain initiates gene expression, which in turn triggers microglia to alter their configuration and function in a "scavenger mode," disposing harmful metabolic products such as amyloid beta and tau with up to a 67% reduction of plaque in mice visual cortex. Furthermore, it may be possible to employ vagal nerve stimulation as well to coax the microglia to perform such functions [11].

The neurobiology of such processes can be attributed to the presence of electrical synapses that dynamically regulate brain networks by virtue of their bidirectionality and continuous properties. Electrical synapses are implicated in the generation of "synchronized neuronal oscillatory activity." Synapses consist of two main configurations, chemical and electrical, with electrical ones using gap junctions allowing bidirectional communication among interconnected cells [12, 13].

An Expedient Quinary System of 5×5 Rules as a Method of Assessment and Management

1. Delineate the clinical diagnostic components into the following:

   (a) Cognitive and behavioral syndromes
   (b) Elementary neurological syndromes
   (c) Neuropsychiatric syndromes
   (d) Cerebrovascular/cardiovascular syndromes
   (e) General medical conditions

2. Follow the multifaceted neuro-investigative approach

   (a) Neuro-laboratory-focused investigation
   (b) Anatomical neuroimaging with multimodality MR imaging
   (c) Functional neuroimaging with fMRI and PET brain scanning
   (d) Cerebrovascular evaluation for small vessel, large vessel, and cardioembolic potential
   (e) Intrinsic connectivity network (ICN) assessment

3. Augmenting brain health and disease-modifying therapies: The 5 brain fitness rules (Fig. 13.3)

   (a) Sleep hygiene
   (b) Brain foods
   (c) Physical exercise

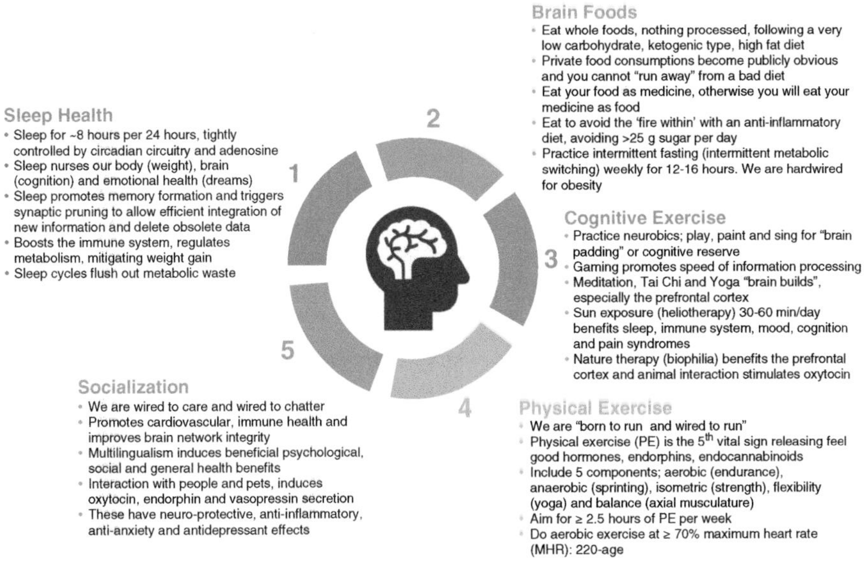

Brain Foods
- Eat whole foods, nothing processed, following a very low carbohydrate, ketogenic type, high fat diet
- Private food consumptions become publicly obvious and you cannot "run away" from a bad diet
- Eat your food as medicine, otherwise you will eat your medicine as food
- Eat to avoid the 'fire within' with an anti-inflammatory diet, avoiding >25 g sugar per day
- Practice intermittent fasting (intermittent metabolic switching) weekly for 12-16 hours. We are hardwired for obesity

Sleep Health
- Sleep for ~8 hours per 24 hours, tightly controlled by circadian circuitry and adenosine
- Sleep nurses our body (weight), brain (cognition) and emotional health (dreams)
- Sleep promotes memory formation and triggers synaptic pruning to allow efficient integration of new information and delete obsolete data
- Boosts the immune system, regulates metabolism, mitigating weight gain
- Sleep cycles flush out metabolic waste

Cognitive Exercise
- Practice neurobics; play, paint and sing for "brain padding" or cognitive reserve
- Gaming promotes speed of information processing
- Meditation, Tai Chi and Yoga "brain builds", especially the prefrontal cortex
- Sun exposure (heliotherapy) 30-60 min/day benefits sleep, immune system, mood, cognition and pain syndromes
- Nature therapy (biophilia) benefits the prefrontal cortex and animal interaction stimulates oxytocin

Socialization
- We are wired to care and wired to chatter
- Promotes cardiovascular, immune health and improves brain network integrity
- Multilingualism induces beneficial psychological, social and general health benefits
- Interaction with people and pets, induces oxytocin, endorphin and vasopressin secretion
- These have neuro-protective, anti-inflammatory, anti-anxiety and antidepressant effects

Physical Exercise
- We are "born to run and wired to run"
- Physical exercise (PE) is the 5th vital sign releasing feel good hormones, endorphins, endocannabinoids
- Include 5 components; aerobic (endurance), anaerobic (sprinting), isometric (strength), flexibility (yoga) and balance (axial musculature)
- Aim for ≥ 2.5 hours of PE per week
- Do aerobic exercise at ≥ 70% maximum heart rate (MHR): 220-age

Fig. 13.3 Brain fitness rules: executive summary

(d) Cognitive exercise

(e) Socialization

4. Major modifying conditions

   (a) Vascular health
   (b) Senotherapeutics
   (c) Gut microbiome
   (d) Exclude deleterious drugs
   (e) Exclude neurotoxicological influence

5. Interventional therapies including neuroplasticity approaches

   (a) Neuropharmacological
   (b) Device therapies – magnetic, electrical, laser ultrasound
   (c) Cognitive behavioral therapy
   (d) Psycho-neurosurgery
   (e) Medical coaching

Vascular Dysregulation (Fig. 13.4)

Vascular dysregulation has been shown to be the earliest finding underlying neuro-degenerative disease, including all the major dementias (Alzheimer's frontotemporal degenerations, Lewy body disease, cognitive vascular, mixed dementia). Following small vessel cerebrovascular disease dysfunction, A-beta deposition follows due to impaired clearance rather than overproduction. Blood–brain barrier (BBB) dysfunction and permeability enable the misfolded protein deposition and subsequent toxicity, which in turn is toxic to the mitochondria with accompanying reactive oxygen species production. Finally, neuronal and glial degeneration leads to clinically apparent cognitive decline and atrophy as confirmed by neuroimaging [14].

Senotherapeutics (Fig. 13.5)

Senescent brain cells have been demonstrated to portray abnormal features, termed "neuronal cell cycle activation," whereby there is a phagocytosis of still viable neurons and synapses mediated by glial cells. This has been linked to microbes interfering with the immune system and initiating neurodegeneration and also to the breakdown of the integrity of biological barriers (gut, BBB). This pathophysiological understanding has led to a number of potential treatment interventions

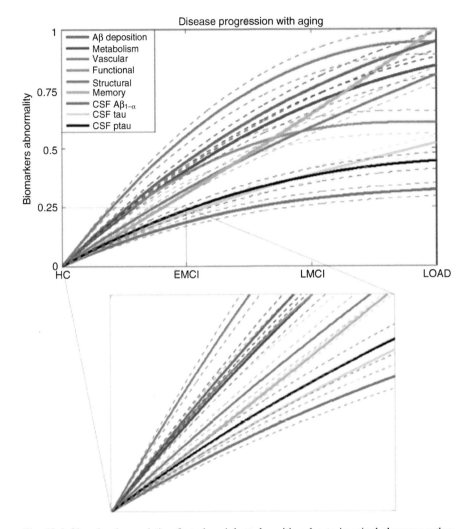

Fig. 13.4 Vascular dysregulation first, then A-beta deposition due to impaired clearance rather than by an A-beta overproduction. The brown line indicates the much earlier vascular dysregulation and the red line the amyloid deposition. (Legend: FIturria-Medina et al. [14])

including inflammasome inhibitors (short chain fatty acids), iron chelators (deferoxamine, lactoferrin), mitophagy (doxycycline, metformin, minocycline), histone deacetylase inhibitors (valproate, sodium butyrate), as well as the possible use of repurposed drugs (donepezil, fluoxetine, lithium). In addition, vagal nerve stimulation and t-DCS have been shown to enhance cholinergic signaling [15].

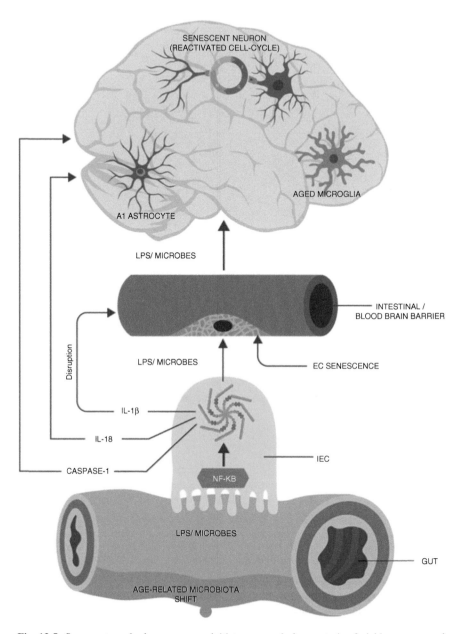

Fig. 13.5 Senescent cerebral neurons may initiate neuronal phagocytosis of viable neurons and synapses by glial cells – inflammasomes. (Figure with permission: Osorio et al. [15])

Gut Microbiome

The gut has a significant role in the regulation of emotional states mediated principally by the vagal sensory neurons stimulating brain-reward neurons. The right sensory vagal ganglion activation, specifically, not left, causes dopamine release from substantia nigra, underscoring the vagal gut-brain axis as an innate component of the neuronal reward circuitry. This has led to implementation of vagal neurostimulation for the treatment for refractory major depression (FDA approved) with positive states more likely induced by stimulating the right vagus nerve [16].

Exclude Deleterious Drugs

Ten major drug categories are responsible for the vast majority of drug-related mental status confusion, altered mental status, and mild cognitive impairment [17] and are as follows:

- Central nervous system medications: hypnotics (benzodiazepines), anticonvulsants (barbiturates), anti-Parkinson's agents such as benztropine and trihexyphenidyl
- Analgesics: narcotics, meperidine, non-steroidal anti-inflammatory agents
- Antihistamines: hydroxyzine
- Gastrointestinal medications: antispasmodics, H-2 blockers
- Anti-nausea agents: scopolamine, dimenhydrinate
- Antibiotics: fluoroquinolones
- Psychotropic medications: tricyclic antidepressants, lithium
- Cardiac medications: antiarrhythmics, digitalis, anti-hypertensives, especially beta blockers and methyldopa
- Others: steroids, muscle relaxants
- Over-the-counter drugs and herbal remedies: antihistamines, medications containing alcohol, mandrake, henbane, Jimson weed

Exclude Neurotoxicological Influence

People who have chronic exposures to solvent, fuel, vapor, or emissions as part of their job are prolific. These include military personal in all branches, hair dressers, painters, dry-wall construction workers, carpenters, mechanics, and laboratory technicians. Mild and at times moderate cognitive impairment is common, and typical features include impaired executive function, working memory, speed of information processing, as well as frequent mild behavioral disorders [18].

Management of the underlying condition or pathophysiological process is key. A good example is autoimmune encephalitis in which treatments such as Intravenous immune globulin (IVIG) or plasmapheresis is curative and may reverse all cognitive and behavioral deficits. This was well illustrated by the true story and movie "Brain on Fire" [19].

The following summarizes treatment approaches in cognitive and behavioral disorders with varying degrees of support from case series, case control trials, and a number of double-blinded randomized control trials.

General Frontal Network Syndrome Remediation

- NeuroRacer custom video game training
- Applied mindfulness – redirection of attention to pertinent goals
- Mindfulness-based attention regulation training – minimize non-relevant information [20] (Fig. 13.6)

Dorsolateral Prefrontal Syndrome Attention Deficit Hyperactivity Disorder, Tourettes Syndrome, Frontotemporal Disorder

- Dopaminergic and noradrenergic therapy [21, 22]
- Idazoxan for frontotemporal degeneration [23]

The Anterior Cingulate syndrome of Apathy and Akinetic Mutism

- Dopaminergic agents, bromocriptine, amantadine, methylphenidate, bupropion [24–28]

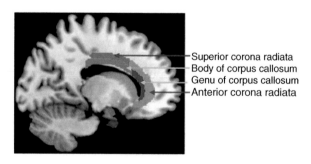

Superior corona radiata
Body of corpus callosum
Genu of corpus callosum
Anterior corona radiata

Fig. 13.6 Meditation "brain builds." White matter connectivity to the anterior cingulate gyrus increases in efficiency and integrity. FA increases (all significant) in the superior corona radiata (purple), body of the corpus callosum (red), genu of the corpus callosum (blue), and left anterior corona radiata (green). (Figure credit with permission: Tang et al. [84])

Medial Orbitofrontal Syndrome, Disinhibition, and Behavioral Abnormalities

- Fluoxetine
- Buspirone, sodium valproate
- Carbamazepine
- Propranolol, pindolol
- Clonidine
- Lithium [29–32]

Lateral Orbitofrontal Syndrome and Obsessive-Compulsive Disorder (OCD)

- Cognitive behavioral therapy
- Selective serotonin reuptake inhibitors (SSRI)
- Combination of both potentiates treatment effect [33]

Frontotemporal Sequelae of TBI (Randomized Controlled Trials)

- Trazodone for frontotemporal lobe disorder (FTLD) [81, 82]
- Amantadine for severe traumatic brain injury (TBI) [34]
- Methylphenidate for moderate to severe TBI [35]
- Serotonergic therapy and stroke (motor deficit) [36]

Depression [37–39, 40]

- Serotonergic agents
- Electroconvulsive therapy
- Transcranial magnetic stimulation
- Physical exercise
- Cognitive behavioral therapy
- Ketamine infusions
- Psychosurgical treatment – anterior cingulotomy for severe treatment-resistant depression (see below)

Attention Deficit Hyperactivity Disorder

- Ketogenic diet
- Methylphenidate
- Atomoxetine [41]

Involuntary Emotional Expression Disorders (IEED) and Emotional Intelligence Impairment

- Dextromethorpan-quinidine combination (Nuedexta) [42, 43]
- Behavioral programs that endeavor to improve one's emotional responses [44–46]

Task-Orientated and Repetitive Training-Based Interventions (Randomized Controlled Trials)

- Attention post-TBI – attentional training: improvement
- Apraxia – apraxia training: improvement

Systematic Reviews

- Aphasia – intensive treatment: improvement based on systemic reviews
- Neglect post-stroke – visual scanning and visuospatial motor training
- Attention disorders post-stroke – attention task improvement
- Memory post-stroke – errorless learning (electronic aids): improvement [47]
- Constraint therapy [48, 49]

Episodic Memory

- Discontinue anticholinergically active medications if possible
- Episodic memory rehabilitation – PQRST method [120]
- Spaced retrieval training – USMART (Ubiquitous Spaced Retrieval-Based Memory Advancement and Rehabilitation Training) [50]
- Vanishing cues (VC) and errorless learning (EL) techniques [51]
- Ecologically orientated neuro-rehabilitation of memory (EON-MEM) [52]

Working Memory (WM) Improvement and Rehabilitation

- Computerized WM training programs [53, 54]
- Working memory improvement facilitated by physical exercise [55, 56]

Apraxia Treatments

- Behavioral training program – gesture-production exercises, with or without symbolic value [57, 58]
- t-DCS with ideomotor apraxia – the Jebsen Hand Function Test [59]
- Gait apraxia – dopamine agonists such as ropinirole [60]

Aphasia Treatment [61–67]

- Intensive speech language aphasia therapy
- Pharmacological (nootropics, dopamine, methylphenidate, donepezil)
- Melodic Intonation Therapy
- Gestural therapy
- Constraint induced therapy for aphasia
- Transcranial Magnetic Stimulation Therapy
- Transcranial direct current stimulation
- Situational therapy for Wernicke's aphasia
- Right hemisphere engagement

Right Hemisphere Neglect management and Treatment Options [68–76]

- Visual scanning training for reducing unilateral spatial neglect
- Mirror therapy for unilateral spatial neglect
- Constraint induced therapy motor therapy (CIMT)
- Directing attention to contra-lesional space
- Cross sensory stimulation techniques – caloric stimulation and optokinetic stimulation
- Music therapy for facilitating, attention, emotion, cognition, behavior, and gait

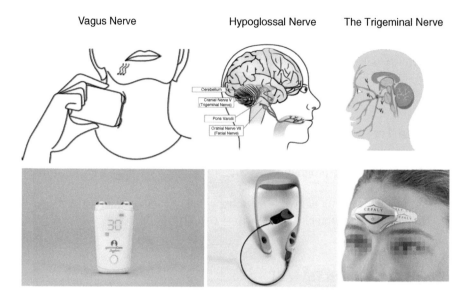

Fig. 13.7 Cranial nerve stimulation devices: GammaCor Sapphire (vagus), PoNS (hypoglossal), Cefaly (trigeminal)

Devices and Minimally Invasive Procedures (Fig. 13.7)

Vagal nerve stimulation has been used to treatment resistant epilepsy and depression with considerable success. More recently, migraine treatment has been added to the list with favorable results. This has led to improvements in other cognitive functions such as executive function and working memory [77, 78]. In view of approximately 80% of the vagal nerve fibers being afferent, linking the peripheral organs to the brain with stimulation engendering a bottom up brainstem stimulation via the nucleus tractus solitarius to the insula and orbitofrontal cortex. The presumed mechanisms include modulation of GABA, serotonin, and norepinephrine, as well as triggering release of brain derived neurotrophic factor (BDNF) [79]. Sphenopalatine ganglion stimulation has been used with success in acute stroke treatment, whereby augmentation of ipsilateral collateral blood flow and stabilization of the blood brain barrier were documented [80].

- Transcranial magnetic stimulation – augmenting hypofunction, inhibiting excitatory effects
- Transcranial direct current stimulation (t-DCS) – speech fluency and stuttering
- Gammacor sapphire - migraine
- PoNS – various neurological syndromes including cognition
- Cefaly – migraine
- Stellate ganglia block – post-traumatic stress disorder
- Sphenopalatine ganglion stimulation – acute stroke blood flow augmentation
- Focused ultrasound for tremor

Psycho-Neurosurgery [81]

Reserved for treatment-resistant conditions, the overall success rate ranges from 40 to 70% for appropriately selected people with ~25% showing exceptional improvement. Currently three different brain regions are routinely targeted by four different neurosurgical ablating procedures, performed by image-based stereotactic guidance:

- Anterior cingulotomy – treatment-resistant depression and obsessive-compulsive disorder (OCD)
- Sub-caudate tractotomy (basal forebrain, substantia innominate) – depression, OCD
- Anterior capsulotomy (anterior limb of internal capsule) – intractable OCD
- Limbic leucotomy (combination of anterior cingulotomy and sub-caudate tactotomy) – depression, OCD
- Deep brain stimulation – Parkinson's, essential tremor, Tourette syndrome, depression

Medical Coaching

Both personal and medical coaching have experienced a major upsurge in popularity. Benefits provided by a personal fitness trainer include motivation, implementation of exercise prescription and monitoring performance indicators. Comparable approaches can be used for the implementation of health coaching. This was well demonstrated by the SAMMPRIS stroke trial where professional coaching of lifestyle adherence achieved remarkable success. This led to a dramatic outcome in favor of the lifestyle and medical treatment arm being markedly superior to the angioplasty and stenting arm for intracranial stenosis [82].

References

1. Xie L, et al. Sleep drives metabolite clearance from the adult brain. Science. 2013;342:373–377 and underwood E. sleep: the Brain's housekeeper? Science. 2013;342:301.
2. Fregni F, Pascual-Leone A. Technology insight: noninvasive brain stimulation in neurology: perspectives on the therapeutic potential of rTMS and tDCS. Nat Clin Pract Neurol. 2007;3:383–93.
3. Lindenberger U, Wenger E, Lövden M. Towards a stronger science of human plasticity. Nat Rev Neurosci. 2017;18:261–2.
4. Cavanaugh MR, Huxlin KR. Visual discrimination training improves Humphrey perimetry in chronic cortically induced blindness. Neurology. 2017;88:1856–64.
5. Stern Y, Mackay-Brandt A, Lee S, et al. Effect of aerobic exercise on cognition in younger adults. A randomized clinical trial. Neurology. 2019:e905–16.
6. Ahlskog JE, Geda YE, Graff-Radford NR, Petersen RC. Physical exercise as a preventive or disease-modifying treatment of dementia and brain aging. Mayo Clin Proc. 2011;86(9):876–84.

7. Ngandu T, Lehtisalo J, Solomon A, et al. A 2-year multidomain intervention of diet, exercise, cognitive training, and vascular risk monitoring versus control to prevent cognitive decline in at-risk elderly people (FINGER): a randomised controlled trial. Lancet. 2015;385:2255–63.
8. Hughes LE, Rittman T, Robbins TW, Rower JB. Reorganization of cortical oscillatory dynamics underlying disinhibition in frontotemporal dementia. Brain. 2018;141:2486–99.
9. Thomson H. Wave therapy. Nature. 2018;555:20–2.
10. Malkani RG, Zee PC. BrainStimulation for improving sleep and memory. Sleep Med Clin. 2020;15(1):101–15.
11. Kaczmarczyk R, Tejera D, Simon BJ, Heneka MT. Microglia modulation through external vagus nerve stimulation in a murine model of Alzheimer's disease. J Neurochem. 2018;146:76. https://doi.org/10.1111/jnc.14284.
12. Alcami P, Pereda AE. Beyond plasticity: the dynamic impact of electrical synapses on neural circuits. Nat Rev Neurosci. 2019;20:253–71.
13. Connors BW. Synchrony and so much more diverse roles for electrical synapses in neural circuits. Dev Neurobiol. 2017;77:610–24.
14. FIturria-Medina Y, Sotero RC, Toussaint PJ et al. Early role of vascular dysregulation on late onset Alzheimer's disease based on multifactorial data driven analysis. Nature Communications 21 June 2016.
15. Osorio C, Kanukuntla T, Diaz E, Jafri N, Cummings M, Sfera A. The post amyloid era in Alzheimer's disease: trust your gut feeling. Front Aging Neurosci. 2019; https://doi.org/10.3389/fnagi.2019.00143.
16. Han W, Tellez LA, Perkins MH, et al. A neural circuit for gut-induced reward. Cell. 2018;175:665–78.
17. Marcantonio ER. Delirium in hospitalized older adults. N Engl J Med. 2017;377:1456–66.
18. Tang CY, Carpenter DM, Eaves EL, et al. Occupational solvent exposure and brain function: an f-MRI study. Environ Health Perspect. 2011;119:908–13.
19. Cahalan S. Brain on fire: my month of madness. New York: Simon and Schuster; 2013.
20. Novakovic-Agopian T, Chen A, Rome AJW, et al. Rehabilitation of executive functioning with training in attention regulation applied to individually defined goals: a pilot study bridging theory, assessment and treatment. J Head Trauma Rehabil. 2011;26:325–38.
21. Arnsten AFT, Goldman Rakic PS. Alpha 2 adrenergic mechanism in prefrontal cortex associated with cognitive decline in aged non human primates. Science. 1985;230:1273–6.
22. Arnsten AFT, Steere JC, Hunt RD. The contribution of alpha 2 noradrenergic mechanisms to prefrontal cortical function: potential significance for attention deficit hyperactivity disorder. Arch Gen Psychiatry. 1995;53:448–55.
23. Sahakian BJ, Coull JJ, Hodges JR. Selective enhancement of executive function by idazoxan in a patient with dementia of the frontal lobe type. J Neurol Neurosurg Pyschiatry. 1994;57:120–1.
24. Marin RS, Fogel BS, Hawkins J, Duffy J, Krupp B, Tolosa E, Zee DS. Apathy: a treatable syndrome. J Neuropsychiatry Clin Neurosci. 1995;7:23–30.
25. Wantanabe MD, Martin EM, DeLeon OA, Gaviria M, Pavel DG, Trepashko DW. Successful methylphenidate treatment of apathy after subcortical infarcts. J Neuropsychiatry Clin Neurosci. 1995;7:502–4.
26. Barrett K. Treating organic abulia with bromocriptine and lisuride: Four studies. J Neurol Neurosurg Pyschiatry. 1991;54:7180721.
27. Holmes VF, Fernandes F, Levy JK. Psychostimulant therapy in AIDS related complex patients. J Clin Psychiatry. 1989;50:5–8.
28. Parks RW, Crockett DJ, Manji HK, Ammann W. Assessment of bromocriptine intervention for the treatment of frontal lobe syndrome: a case study. J Neuropsychiatry Clin Neurosci. 1992;4:109–11.
29. Hollander E, Wong CM. Body dysmorphic disorder, pathological gambling, and sexual compulsions. J Clin Psychiatry. 1995;56:7–12.
30. Olivier B, Mos J. Serenics and aggression. Stress Med. 1986;2:197–209.
31. Bakchine S, Lacomblez L, Benoit N, Parisot D, Chain F, Lhermitte F. Manic-like state after bilateral orbitofrontal and right temporoparietal injury: efficacy of clonidine. Neurology. 1989;39:777–81.

32. Tariot PN, Schneider LS, Cummings J, Thomas RG, Raman R, Jakimovich LJ, Loy R, Bartocci B, Fleisher A, Ismail MS, Porsteinsson A, Weiner M, Jack CR Jr, Thal L, Aisen PS. Chronic divalproex sodium to attenuate agitation and clinical progression of Alzheimer disease.; Alzheimer's disease cooperative study group. Arch Gen Psychiatry. 2011;68:853–61.

33. O'Connor K, Todorov C, Robillard S, Borgeat F, Brault M. Cognitive-behaviour therapy and medication in the treatment of obsessive-compulsive disorder: a controlled study. Can J Psychiatr. 1999;44:64–71.

34. Giacino JT, Whyte J, Bagiella E, Kalmar K, Childs N, Khademi A, Eifert B, Long D, Katz DI, Cho S, Yablon SA, Luther M, Hammond FM, Nordenbo A, Novak P, Mercer W, Maurer-Karattup P, Sherer M. Placebo-controlled trial of amantadine for severe traumatic brain injury. N Engl J Med. 2012;366:819–26.

35. Willmott C, Ponsford J. Efficacy of methylphenidate in the rehabilitation of attention following traumatic brain injury: a randomised, crossover, double blind, placebo controlled inpatient trial. J Neurol Neurosurg Psychiatry. 2009;80:552–7.

36. Chollet F, Tardy J, Albucher JF, Thalamas C, Berard E, Lamy C, Bejot Y, Deltour S, Jaillard A, Niclot P, Guillon B, Moulin T, Marque P, Pariente J, Arnaud C, Loubinoux I. Fluoxetine for motor recovery after acute ischaemic stroke (FLAME): a randomised placebo-controlled trial. Lancet Neurol. 2011;10:123–30.

37. Rimer J, Dwan K, Lawlor DA, Greig CA, McMurdo M, Morley W, Mead GE. Exercise for depression. Cochrane Database Syst Rev. 2012;7:CD004366.

38. Lee JC, Blumberger DM, Fitzgerald P, Daskalakis Z. Levinson a The Role of Transcranial Magnetic Stimulation in Treatment-Resistant Depression: A Review. Curr Pharm Des. 2012;6. [Epub ahead of print]

39. Farahani A, Correll CU. Are antipsychotics or antidepressants needed for psychotic depression? A systematic review and meta-analysis of trials comparing antidepressant or antipsychotic monotherapy with combination treatment. J Clin Psychiatry. 2012;73(4):486–96.. Review

40. Dougherty DD, Weiss AP, Cosgrove GR, Alpert NM, Cassem EH, Nierenberg AA, Price BH, Mayberg HS, Fischman AJ, Rauch SL. Cerebral metabolic correlates as potential predictors of response to anterior cingulotomy for treatment of major depression. J Neurosurg. 2003;99:1010–7.

41. Chamberlain SR, Del Campo N, Dowson J, Muller U, Clark L, et al. Atomoxetine improved response inhibition in adults with attention deficit hyperactivity disorder. Biol Pyschiatry. 2007;62:977–84.

42. Panitch HS, Thisted RA, Smith RA, Wynn DR, Wymer JP, Achiron A, Vollmer TL, Mandler RN, Dietrich DW, Fletcher M, Pope LE, Berg JE, Miller A. Pseudobulbar affect in multiple sclerosis study group. Ann Neurol. 2006;59:780–7.

43. Miller A, Pratt H, Schiffer RB. Pseudobulbar affect: the spectrum of clinical presentations, etiologies and treatments. Expert Rev Neurother. 2011;11:1077–88.

44. Davidson RJ, Begley S. In their book the emotional life of your brain. New York: Hudson Street Press; 2012.

45. Fava GA, Tomba E. Increasing psychological Well-being and resilience by psychotherapeutic methods. J Pers. 2009;77:1903–34.

46. Hoelzel BK, Ott U, Gard T, Hempel H, Weygandt M, Morgen K, Vaitl D. Investigation of mindfulness meditation practitioners with voxel based morphometry. Soc Cogn Affect Neurosci. 2008;3:55–61.

47. Cappa SF, Benke T, Clarke S, Rossi B, Stemmer B, van Heugten CM. EFNS guidelines on cognitive rehabilitation: report of an EFNS task force. Eur Neurol. 2005;12:665–80.

48. Wolf SL, Winstein CJ, Miller JP, Taub E, Uswatte G, Morris D, Giuliani C, Light KE, Nichols-Larsen DS. Effect of constraint induced movement therapy on upper extremity function 3 to 9 months after stroke: the EXCITE randomized clinical trial. JAMA. 2006;296:2095–104.

49. Wolf SL, Thompson PA, Winstein CJ, Miller JP, Blanton SR, Nichols-Larsen DS, Morris DM, Uswatte G, Taub E, Light KE, Swaki L. The EXCITE stroke trial: comparing early and delayed constraint induced movement therapy. Stroke. 2010;41:2309–15.

50. Han JW, Oh K, Yoo S, et al. Development of the ubiquitous spaced retrieval-based memory advancement and rehabilitation training program. Psychiatry Investig. 2014;11(1):52–8.
51. Haslam C, Moss Z, Hodder K. Are two methods better than one? Evaluating the effectiveness of combining errorless learning with vanishing cues. J Clin Exp Neuropsychol. 2010;32(9):973–85.
52. Stringer AY, Small SK. Ecologically-oriented neurorehabilitation of memory: robustness of outcome across diagnosis and severity. Brain Inj. 2011;25(2):169–78.
53. Klingberg T, et al. Training of working memory in children with ADHD. J Clin Exp Neuropsychol. 2002;24:781–91.
54. Klingberg T, et al. Computerized training of working memory in children with ADHD – a randomized controlled trial. J Am Acad Child Adolesc Psychiatry. 2005;44:177–86.
55. Sibley BA, Beilock SL. Exercise and working memory: an individual differences investigation. J Sport Exerc Psychol. 2007;29:783–91.
56. Zhu N, Jacobs DR, Schreiner PJ, Yaffe K, Bryan N, Launer LJ, Whitmer RA, Sidney S, Demerath E, Thomas W, Bouchard C, He K, Reis J, Sternfeld B. Cardiorespiratory fitness and cognitive function in middle age. CARDIA Study Neurol. 2014;82:1339–46.
57. Smania N, Girardi F, Domenicali C, Lora E, Aglioti S. The rehabilitation of limb apraxia: a study in left-brain-damaged patients. Arch Phys Med Rehabil. 2000;81(4):379–88.
58. Bolognini N, Convento S, Banco E, Mattioli F, Tesio L, Vallar G. Improving ideomotor limb apraxia by electrical stimulation of the left parietal cortex. Brain. 2015;138:428–39.
59. Bianchi M, Cosseddu M, Cotelli M, Manenti R, Brambilla M, Rizzetti MC, Padovani A, Borroni B. Left parietal cortex transcranial direct current stimulation enhances gesture processing in corticobasal syndrome. Eur J Neurol. 2015;22:1317. https://doi.org/10.1111/ene.12748.
60. Taskapilioglu O, Karli N, Erer S, Zarifoglu M, Bakar M, Turan F. Primary gait ignition disorder: report of three cases. Neurol Sci. 2009;30:333–7.
61. Raymer AM, McHose B, Smith KG, Iman L, Ambrose A, Casselton C. Contrasting effects of errorless naming treatment and gestural facilitation for word retrieval in aphasia. Neuropsychol Rehabil. 2012;22(2):235–66.
62. Hanlon Brown RE, Brown JW, Gerstman LJ. Enhancement of naming in nonfluent aphasia through gesture. Brain Lang. 1990;38:298–314.
63. Hadar U, Wenkert-Olenik D, Krauss R, Soroker N. Gesture and processing of speech: neuropsychological evidence. Brain Lang. 1998;62:107–26.
64. Garrison KA, et al. The mirror neuron system: a neural substrate for methods in stroke rehabilitation. Neurorehabil Neural Repair. 2010;5:404–12.
65. Bonilha L, Gleichgerrcht E, Nesland T, Rorden C, Fridriksson J. Success of Anomia Treatment in Aphasia Is Associated With Preserved Architecture of Global and Left Temporal Lobe Structural Networks. Neurorehabil Neural Repair. 2015;. pii: 1545968315593808
66. Altschuler EL, Multari A, Hirstein W, Ramachandran VS. Situational therapy for Wernicke's aphasia. Med Hypotheses. 2006;67(4):713–6.
67. Pulvermüller F, Roth VM. Communicative aphasia treatment as a further development of PACE therapy. Aphasiology. 1991;5:39–5.
68. Corbetta M. Hemispatial neglect: clinic, pathogenesis, and treatment. Semin Neurol. 2014;34(5):514–23.
69. Matano A, Iosa M, Guariglia C, Pizzamiglio L, Paolucci S. Does outcome of neuropsychological treatment in patients with unilateral spatial neglect after stroke affect functional outcome? Eur J Phys Rehabil Med. 2015;51:737–43.
70. Pandian JD, Arora R, Kaur P, et al. Mirror therapy in unilateral neglect after stroke (MUST trial): a randomized controlled trial. Neurology. 2014;83(11):1012–7.
71. Arai T, Ohi H, Sasak H, Nobuto H, Tanaka K. Heimspatial sunglasses: effect on unilateral spatial neglect. Archiv Phys Med Rehabil. 1997;78:230–2.

72. Gorgoraptis N, Mah YH, Machner B, et al. The effects of the dopamine agonist rotigotine on hemispatial neglect following stroke. Brain. 2012;135(Pt 8):2478–91.
73. Buxbaum LJ, Ferraro M, Whyte J, Gershkoff A, Coslett HB. Amantadine treatment of hemispatial neglect: a double-blind, placebo-controlled study. Am J Phys Med Rehabil. 2007;86(7):527–37.
74. Jacquin-Courtois S. Hemi-spatial neglect rehabilitation using non-invasive brain stimulation: Or how to modulate the disconnection syndrome? Ann Phys Rehabil Med. 2015. pii: S1877–0657(15)00471–6; https://doi.org/10.1016/j.rehab.2015.07.388.
75. Goedert KM, Zhang JY, Barrett AM. Prism adaptation and spatial neglect: the need for dose-finding studies. Front Hum Neurosci. 2015;9:243. https://doi.org/10.3389/fnhum.2015.00243.. eCollection 2015
76. Guilbert A, Clément S, Moroni C. Hearing and music in unilateral spatial neglect neuro-rehabilitation. Front Psychol. 2014;5:1503. https://doi.org/10.3389/fpsyg.2014.01503.
77. Sanders TH, Weiss J, Hogewood L, et al. Cognition-enhancing Vagus nerve stimulation alters the epigenetic landscape. J Neurosci. 2019;39:3454–69.
78. Broncel A, Brocian R, Klos-Woitczak P, et al. Vagal nerve stimulation as a promising tool in the improvement of cognitive disorders. Brain Res Bull. 2020;155:37–47. https://doi.org/10.1016/j.brainresbull.2019.11.011.. Epub 2019
79. O'Reardon JP, Cristancho P, Peshek AD. Vagus nerve stimulation and treatment of depression: to the brainstem and beyond. Psychiatry. 2006;3(5):54–63.
80. Khurana D, et al. ImpACT 1 study group. Implant for augmentation of cerebral blood flow trial 1: a pilot study. Int J Stroke. 2009;4:480–5.
81. Ducharme S, Dougherty DD, Price BH. Neurosurgical treatmetns for psychiatric disorders. In: Miller C, editor. The human frontal lobes. London: Guilford Press; 2018.
82. Turan TN, Nizam A, Lynn MJ, et al. Relationship between risk factor control and vascular events in the SAMMPRIS trial. Neurology. 2017;88:379–85.
83. Ramachandran VS, Altschuler EL. The use of visual feedback, in particular mirror visual feedback, in restoring **brain** function. Brain. 2009;132:1693–710.
84. Tang Y-Y, Lu Q, Gen X, Stein EA, Yang Y, Posner MI. Short-term meditation induces white matter changes in the anterior cingulate. PNAS. 2010;107:15649–15,652.

Chapter 14
Who Needs Evaluation, How, and When? The Case for You, Leaders, Executives, and People in Public Office

Evaluation of cognitive function or assessment of mentation in those with symptoms, or reported by friends or family, has many challenges. A particularly flexible approach is required, as some people cannot even be assessed due to obtundation, some cannot concentrate for more than a few seconds in the case of delirium, and some are inattentive with only minutes of assessment possible (dementias). Extensive in-depth neuropsychological testing at the other extreme is taxing even for normal people. Furthermore, examination technique may be prone to error and misinterpretation, by many factors, including medications (the ubiquitous anticholinergic drug effects) and organ system failure (minimal hepatic encephalopathy). In addition, overdiagnosis of cognitive deficits is not uncommon, even by experienced neuropsychologists [1].

What about people without complaints? Subjective cognitive impairment includes people often described as the "worried well," who usually do not advance to significant cognitive impairment or dementia. However, preclinical Alzheimer's disease is a valid conception even when biomarkers such as CSF amyloid and tau are normal [2].

Estimates from state mandated prevention of medical error courses and psychological reviews, reveal that we all make between 1–2 dozen daily mistakes including memory, calculation and word finding lapses [3]. There are many potential reasons for this (Fig. 14.1). Most notable is a neurobiological reason – we are designed to make a certain number of mistakes as our brain wiring has been programmed to be more concerned with understanding concepts rather than to rote learn. From a paleoneurological point of view, the earliest evidence we have of our species contracting out memorizing vast factual data dates back to about 70,000 years, where ochre engravings may have signified lunar or tidal cycles [4]. We continued to do so ever since, nowadays with terabyte storage capacity available on our laptops. Our brains are designated knowledge organizers and understand information as opposed to data storage devices. Answering the "why" question relating to information we obtain is most important, and from this follows the generation of concepts which requires a stimulus free space. These cerebral processes require quality sleep,

© Springer Nature Switzerland AG 2020
M. Hoffmann, *Clinical Mentation Evaluation*,
https://doi.org/10.1007/978-3-030-46324-3_14

Fig. 14.1 The spectrum from normalcy to illness

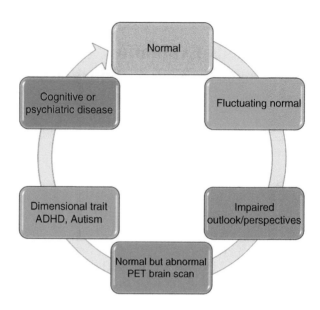

essential for forming brain circuitry, and integration with existing networks. Factors countering this integration include inattention, anxiety, and medications [5].

Normalcy Overlaps with Incipient Clinical Neurological and Neuropsychiatric Syndromes

Our heritage of bipedalism and our extensive tertiary association cortex brain design and emotional circuitry dates to our sojourn on the African savannah over the last 6–seven million years. Clinical experience has long been aware that there are continua between many cognitive and behavioral neurological conditions and normalcy. Likewise, continua are known to be present between normalcy and psychosis, depression and anxiety disorders, delusional disorders and obsessive-compulsive disorder, as well as schizophrenia and bipolar disorder. From a clinical and neurobiological perspective, there is mounting evidence that categorically distinct illness entities for psychiatric syndromes (DSM V, ICD) are not consistent with known neurobiological principles. Some researchers have termed these atheoretical, and that the categorical approach be abandoned and replaced with a so-called "dimensional" approach which is based on etiological and genetic factors. Furthermore, behavior that is viewed as dysfunctional or harmful to the person nowadays in our environment may be entirely functional and beneficial in another (e.g., ADHD and autism). With ADHD, from an evolutionary point of view, upregulated motor activity, explorative behavior, hypervigilance, and attention shifting would have been desired adaptive behavioral traits in potentially dangerous and unpredictable environmental conditions. With autism, men have superior cognitive functions with abilities such as mental rotation, spatial orientation, and physical problem-solving but with relative deficits in social attributes. Hence, autism may present an extreme example of the "male brain traits." Chronic social anxiety may be viewed as a beneficial trait for reminding us of our social status and depression as a type of appeasement or avoiding strategy when faced with socially competitive challenges [6]. Reynolds has a particularly apt summary of these principles akin to the rules of bird-flocking behaviors:

- Stay close together (panic anxiety)
- Follow the crowd (social anxiety)
- Don't crowd your neighbor (atypical depression rejection sensitivity) [7]

The tip of the iceberg phenomenon may be applied to the cognitive, behavioral, and neuropsychiatric conditions, in that all have subclinical variants that may evade casual or at times even deliberate detection (Fig. 14.2). This is underscored by the common news headlines referring to "Why We Snap," also the title of a notable book on this topic [8]. For example, a randomized controlled trial documented ≥30% violence reduction (video surveillance) in young prisoners, achieved with essential fatty acids (EFAs) and micronutrients. It may be surmised too that such behaviors may be a factor in the exponential rise in mass shootings [9]. Quality of life, impaired mental health, and frank psychiatric disorders are all correlated with chronic physical disease such as diabetes, cardiovascular disease, and cancer. Nutrition influences medical syndromes, mental disorders, and mental outlook, and poor physical health is a strong predictor of adverse mental health. The global epidemic of depression, currently 322 million, will be the leading global health problem by 2030. Depression and anxiety already account for ~1/3 of primary care visits and both are upstream and downstream drivers of chronic disease [10].

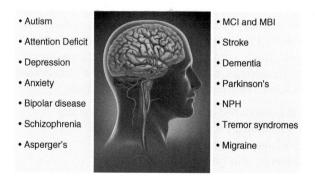

- Autism
- Attention Deficit
- Depression
- Anxiety
- Bipolar disease
- Schizophrenia
- Asperger's

- MCI and MBI
- Stroke
- Dementia
- Parkinson's
- NPH
- Tremor syndromes
- Migraine

Fig. 14.2 The brain, mind, and body do not differentiate between neurological and psychiatric conditions. The cerebrovascular system, nutrition, and microbiome all influence these conditions. Legend: *MCI* mild cognitive impairment, *MBI* mild behavioral impairment, *NPH* normal pressure hydrocephalus

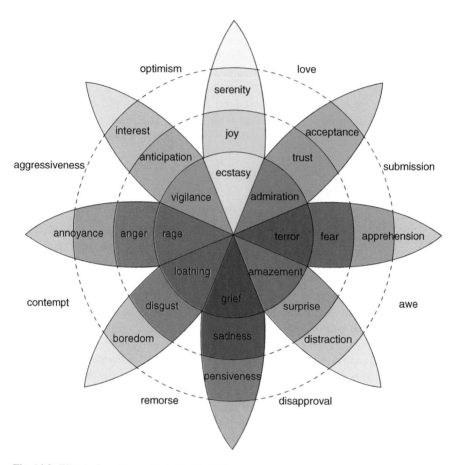

Fig. 14.3 Wheel of emotions. (Plutchik [11, 26])

The many subclinical variants of the panoply of brain syndromes that may be evading our detection may be understood in terms of the concept of mild or partial emotions diagram by Plutchnik (Fig. 14.3) [11]. In addition to the chronic disease and poor physical health, even so-called normal people are subject to the vicissitudes of daily living, and this may significantly affect the brain circuitry manifesting subtle or not-so subtle behavioral vacillation and conditions:

1. Physiological network fluctuations of the prefrontal cortex
2. Physiological hormonal fluctuations
3. Executive entitlement and the fraud triangle
4. Hyperdopaminergic imperatives and personalities
5. Brilliance and baggage

The uniquely sensitive prefrontal cortex (PFC) is concerned with a "top-down" control of thought, emotion, and behavior, a relatively recently acquired circuitry in our evolution. However, these networks are particularly vulnerable to stress, depression, post-traumatic stress disorder, substance abuse, schizophrenia, as well as sleep

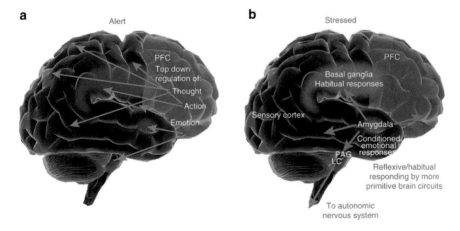

Fig. 14.4 Stress flips the brain from reflective to reflexive behavior. (Arnsten [27])

deprivation. The newly evolved prefrontal pyramidal cell circuitry constitutes the most capricious part of our brain and the apex of our cognitive abilities. With rampant stress, higher cognition is impaired and more primitive amygdala-based cerebral responses occur, switching from a reflective to reflexive brain state. The evolutionary explanation for this capability is of course survival value in context of danger [12] (Fig. 14.4). Decision-making in our daily lives rests on the integrity and proficiency of our prefrontal cortex, most notably the frontopolar cortex (BA 10). Testosterone levels in male traders in the London Stock Exchange affected the rationality of stock market transactions, with elevated levels testosterone correlated with profitability, economic return, and an inflation of the markets, but with increased risk taking. Elevated cortisol was associated with risk aversion, downtrending, and market plunges [13].

Executive entitlement refers to the observation in some that with appointment to supervisor levels, certain individuals develop a misconceived notion of immunity to rules that apply to others [14].

The dopaminergic mind was forged by our prior environmental and societal challenges and evolved circuitry that has addictive components and became very adaptive in coping with uncertainties and psychological stresses of our modern lives. A concept proposed by Fred Previc, the dopaminergic imperative or the dopaminergic personality (impulsiveness, novelty seeking, schizotypal, exploitiveness, far sightedness, motivation for wealth accumulation, restlessness) is useful in understanding what drives some to achieve great feats in human history. Alexander the Great, Einstein, and Newton are some examples. Personal goals also have their downside such as losing approximately a million soldiers' lives by Napoleon's desire to conquer Russia. Relinquishing the Dopamine (DA) imperative may be important to temper in some [15]. Dopamine became the dominant neurotransmitter in humans, and many other conditions can be ascribed to excess imbalance of dopamine (Fig. 14.5).

Akin to schizophrenia and creativity observations is the concept of certain advanced capabilities keeping company with significant other prefrontal

Fig. 14.5 Hyper-
dopaminergic syndromes

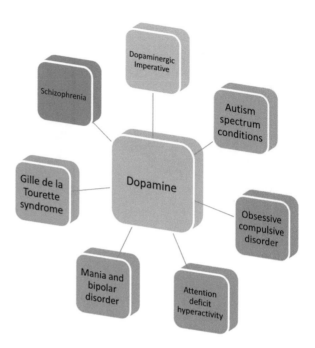

impairment as seen with Asperger's individuals and bipolar disorders among others [16]. Alan Turing was one of the most influential people in the past 100 years, founder of artificial intelligence and computer science. By being able to crack the German naval cryptanalysis codes, it has been estimated that his deliberations shortened WW II in Europe by ~2 years and saved ~14 million lives [17]. He was regarded as having Asperger's syndrome [18]. This has been termed brilliance (the supremely creative traits) and baggage (the associated deleterious traits) by the author and especially well depicted in the accompanying 2014 movie "The Imitation Game."

What Most People Strive For

Most people strive to live long, to live well, and to age with their minds intact. Data from Schwartz et al. revealed that if we are in good physical health, the longer we live, the relatively happier we become continuing until our eigth or ninth decade [19]. The lowest levels of happiness or the nadir occurred in people in their 1950s (Fig.14.6) [20].

Live Well, Feel Well, Lead Well

Appropriate lifestyle adherence needs to be a foundational objective in preventing, ameliorating, and treating not only neurological diseases but also mental resilience

Fig. 14.6 Self-reported
well-being on a
scale of 1–10

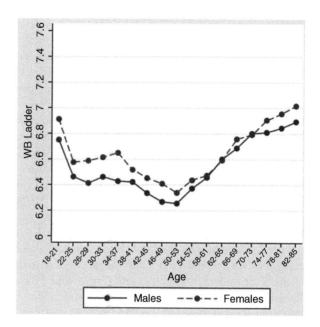

and optimistic disposition. Not only neuropsychiatric illness but also the more commonly encountered behavioral and more subtle manifestations of mild behavioral
impairment stand to be mitigated. Even more covert may be the effects of suboptimal brain health on cognitive flexibility, tenacity, and emotional regulation that can
translate into an aptitude to influence, lead, and be an example to others. To live well
is a prerequisite for peak cognitive function as well as emotional intelligence capacity. The latter is required to lead well. In essence, this is encompassed by the project
"Live Well, Feel Well, Lead Well."

The evidence for promoting such lifestyle adaptations is extensive and compel-
ling. Vascular disease and the metabolic syndrome may be viewed as the primary
manifestations of an unhealthy lifestyle that in turn leads to stroke, the five major
dementias groups, mild cognitive impairment, mild behavioral impairment, and
neuropsychiatric disease. The high-cost hubs of the brain networks, subserving
higher order cognition, are the most vulnerable to metabolic disease and vascular
disease and have been shown to be involved in most, if not all, neurological disease.
Furthermore, the WHO data indicate that ~80% of all cases of cardiovascular disease and type 2 diabetes mellitus and ~ 40% of cancers can potentially be prevented
by adherence to three pillars of healthy living. In addition, mental health syndromes,
most notably depression, affect ~450 million people globally, and present-day estimates are ~873,000 suicides annually. Depression is currently the leading cause of
lost Disability adjusted life years (DALY)s in the world. Given these figures of
epidemic proportions, the manifestation of burnout and other behavioral ill effects
may be viewed as the tip of the iceberg type of phenomenon.

A rapid and easy to follow program for clinicians and patients is presented. This
encompasses "5 key brain fitness rules," detailing not only on (i) "how" to follow

and implement these but also on how to address the underlying (ii) "why" question of the fundamental evolution of our body's requirements for healthy living. The 5 brain fitness rules include physical exercise, cognitive exercises, brain food components, sleep hygiene, and socialization (Chap. 13, Fig. 13.3). An understanding of the "why" factor has repeatedly been shown to promote success in abiding with the recommendations. The third component addresses (iii) key performance indicators both for the patient self-monitoring and for physician-related monitoring indicators. Most of these can be monitored by electronic devices, such as the Garmin VO_2 max for fitness and MUSE meditation monitoring, for example. The fourth component promotes (iv) coaching that at times may spell the difference between success and failure. The fifth component relates to the concept of (v) building cognitive reserve (brain padding) as a buffer against brain aging and disease. Recent data has indicated that ~35% of Alzheimer's disease risk associates with beneficial lifestyle adherence, translating into higher cognitive reserve, leading up to a 40% reduction in dementia. A sixth component of which we should take note and aspire to take a leading role for our profession and subspecialty is that (vi) several international endeavors are underway in this regard. The pivotal Finnish FINGER study powerfully demonstrated that multidomain intervention with physical exercise, cognitive stimulation and high fat, and low carbohydrate nutrition significantly curbs cognitive decline. A groundswell of similar studies has now been adopted in many countries including North America (POINTER study), Asia (SINGER study), Australia (MYB study) Europe (MIND-AD study), and China (MIND-CHINA).

Discerning Brain and Mind Competence in Leaders, CEOs, and Federal Officials

Arias et al. drew attention to this important yet neglected issue [21]. Several other key areas require consideration when ascertaining cerebral competence amongst people in office, or those that may make enduring decisions affecting the public. At the time of writing (2020), even though we currently have the oldest president on record and an increasing number of elderly congress persons, the mean present-day age of Nobel Prize laureates is 72 years. This can be interpreted that perhaps a significant proportion of highly educated people are only peaking in the eighth decade. Furthermore, mild cognitive impairment is well established but mild behavioral impairment much less so, with the latter more often escaping the label of "impaired." The Mini-Mental Sate Examination (MMSE) and Montreal Cognitive Assessment (MOCA) are insensitive to highly educated people, with the former having no frontal function assessment and the latter minimal. The Frontal Assessment Battery does a better job but has no frontal behavioral interrogation of note [22]. To diagnose the extensive repertoire of behavioral syndromes tests such as the Frontal Systems Behavioral Evaluations, Frontal Behavioral Inventory are required, in addition to criteria such as those of Rascovsky and Daphne used for frontotemporal syndrome (FTS) detection. Some are relatively subtle only manifesting in certain situations and these "stealth" FTS are particularly likely to evade the radar of even in-depth neuropsychological examination [23]. In addition, cognitive reserve bolstered by protracted education may be only reliably diagnosed by functional imaging such as metabolic PET scanning.

Research into our global obesity epidemic indicates that there is a close relationship between impaired brain function and elevated body mass index. The most proximal cause is small vessel cerebrovascular disease pathology, now regarded as the underlying pathophysiology in all 5 major groups of dementias [24]. Being physically unfit correlates with being cognitively unfit; an unfit body equals an unfit mind. The good news is that this is potentially mitigated or even reversible. The Norwegian Institute of Technology protocol of "Fitness Age" is an easily computed clinical tool (www.ntnu.edu/cerg/vo2max) that can quantify biological age and allow performance measurements [25]. Other professions that involve substantial societal responsibility, such as commercial pilots and the branches of the military, provide a precedent for requiring medical and cognitive assessments to assure professional competence. Elected officials currently have no such formal protocols. The solution may involve not only deliberate and comprehensive assessment of the wide varieties of behavioral neurological syndromes but also a formal assessment of biological age, in addition to chronological age.

Recommendation of Cognitive and Behavioral Tests for Executives, Leaders, Federal Officials, and You

A. Screening

- COBE 50

B. Cognitive domains

- CNS-VS Subtests

  (a) Speed of information processing
  (b) Working memory tests
  (c) Verbal and visual memory tests
  (d) Executive function tests
  (e) Disinhibition tests
  (f) Perception of Emotions Test

C. Behavioral neurological domains

- Emotional Intelligence Test (Baron)
- Frontal Systems Behavioral Evaluation (FRSBE)
- Frontal Behavioral Inventory (FBI)

D. Neuropsychiatric

- Depression subtests (CNS-VS)
- Anxiety subtest (CNS-VS)
- Obsessive compulsive disorder subtest (CNS-VS)

- Resting state functional connectivity efficiency is predictive of cognitive performance
- Human intellectual performance correlates to how efficiently the brain integrates information amongst disparate brain regions

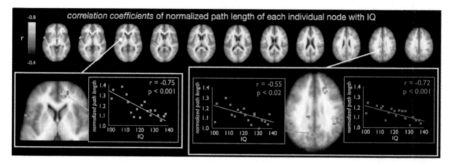

Fig. 14.7 Efficiency of functional brain networks and intellectual performance. (Van den Heuvel et al. [28])

E. Physical exercise measured by "Fitness Age" (www.ntnu.edu/cerg/vo2max)

The ultimate objective is to attain peak network efficiency which correlates with optimum intellectual performance. This in turn translates into the ability to lead well by living well and feeling well (Fig. 14.7).

References

1. Faust D, Guilmette TJ, Hart K, et al. Neuropsychologists' training, experience, and judgment accuracy. Arch Clin Neuropsychol. 1988;3:145–63.
2. Jack CR. Preclinical Alzheimer's disease: a valid concept. Lancet Neurol. 2019;19:31.
3. Mohamed SMH, Börger NA, Geuze RH, van der Meer JJ. Error monitoring and daily life executive functioning. Exp Brain Res. 2019;237:2217–29.
4. Henshilwood CS, d'Errico F, Watts I. Engraved ochres from the Middle Stone Age levels at Blombos Cave, South Africa. J Hum Evol. 2009;57(1):27–47.
5. Scatterbrain BH. How the Mind's mistakes make humans creative, innovative and successful. Vancouver/Berkeley: Greystone Books; 2019.
6. Kahn JP. Angst. Origins of anxiety and depression. New York: Oxford University Press; 2012.
7. Reynolds CW. Flocks, herds and schools: A distributed behavior model. In: Proceedings of the 14th annual conference on computer graphics and interactive 1987.
8. Fields RD. Why we snap. Understanding the rage circuits in your brain. New York: Dutton, Penguin House; 2015.
9. Gesch CB, Hammond SM, Hampson SE, Eves A, Crowder MJ. Influence of supplementary vitamins, minerals and essential fatty acids on the antisocial behavior of young adult prisoners: a randomized placebo-controlled trial. Br J Psychiatry. 2002;181:22–228.
10. Bijl RV, de Graaf R, Hiripi E, Kessler RC, Kohn R, Offord DR, Ustun TB, Vicente B, Vollebergh WA, Walters EE, Wittchen HU. The prevalence of treated and untreated mental disorders in five countries. Health Aff. 2003;22:122–33.
11. Plutchik R. Emotions and life: perspectives from psychology, biology, and evolution. Washington, DC: American Psychological Association; 2002.

12. AFT A. Loss of Prefrontal Cortical Higher Cognition with Uncontrollable Stress: Molecular Mechanisms, Changes with Age, and Relevance to Treatment. Brain Sci. 2019;9:113. https://doi.org/10.3390/brainsci9050113.

13. Coates JM, Herbert J. Endogenous steroids and financial risk taking on a London trading floor. PNAS. 2008;105:6167–72.

14. Wagoner Downing L. www.ACFE.com.

15. Previc FH. The dopaminergic mind in human evolution and history. New York: Cambridge University Press; 2009.

16. Carson S. Schizophrenia hypothesis: creativity and eccentricity. Scientific American Mind May/June 2011.

17. Richelson JT. A century of spies: intelligence in the twentieth century. New York: Oxford University Press; 1997. He was regarded as having Asperger's syndrome

18. O'Connell H, Fitzgerald M. Did Alan Turing have Asperger's syndrome? Ir J Psychol Med. 2003;20:28–31.

19. Stone AA, Schwartz JE, Broderick JE, Deaton A. A snapshot of the age distribution of psychological well-being in the United States.

20. Nielsen, Merrill Lynch data.

21. Arias JJ, Stephens ML, Rabinovici GD. Legal and policy challenges to addressing cognitive impairment in Federal Officials. JAMA Neurol. 2019;4: 392. Published online Feb.

22. Dubois B, Slachevsky A, Litvan I, Pillon B, The FAB. A frontal assessment battery at the beside. Neurology. 2000;55:1621–6.

23. Lhermitte F. Human autonomy and the frontal lobes. Part II: patient behavior in complex and social situations: the "environmental dependency syndrome". Ann Neurol. 1986;19:335–43.

24. Raz L, Knoefel J, Bhaskar K. The neuropathology and cerebrovascular mechanisms of dementia. J Cereb Blood Flow Metab. 2015;36:172. https://doi.org/10.1038/jcbfm.2015.164.

25. Nauman J, Nes BM, Lavie CJ, et al. Prediction of cardiovascular mortality by estimated cardiorespiratory fitness independent of traditional risk factors: the HUNT study. Mayo Clin Proc. 2017;92(2):218–27.

26. Plutchik R. Emotion: Theory, research, and experience: Vol. 1. Theories of emotion 1. New York: Academic; 1980.

27. Arnsten AF. Stress weakens prefrontal networks: molecular insults to higher cognition. Nat Neurosci. 2015;18:1376–85.

28. Van den Heuvel MP, Stam CJ, Kahn RS, Hulshoff Pol HE. Efficiency of functional brain networks and intellectual performance. J Neurosci. 2009;29:7619–24.

Index

© Springer Nature Switzerland AG 2020
M. Hoffmann, *Clinical Mentation Evaluation*,
https://doi.org/10.1007/978-3-030-46324-3

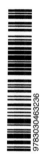